Change Your
FOOD
Change Your
MOOD

JANET
MACCARO, PhD, CNC

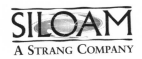

SILOAM

A STRANG COMPANY

Most Strang Communications/Charisma House/Siloam/FrontLine/Realms/Excel Books products are available at special quantity discounts for bulk purchase for sales promotions, premiums, fund-raising, and educational needs. For details, write Strang Communications/Charisma House/Siloam/FrontLine/Realms/Excel Books, 600 Rinehart Road, Lake Mary, Florida 32746, or telephone (407) 333-0600.

Change Your Food, Change Your Mood
by Janet Maccaro, PhD, CNC
Published by Siloam
A Strang Company
600 Rinehart Road
Lake Mary, Florida 32746
www.siloam.com

Unless otherwise noted, Scripture quotations are from the New American Standard Bible, Updated. Copyright © 1960, 1962, 1963, 1968, 1971, 1972, 1973, 1975, 1977, 1995 by the Lockman Foundation. Used by permission (www.Lockman.org).

Cover Designer: Judith McKittrick
Executive Design Director: Bill Johnson
Author Photo: Markow Southwest, www.paul.markow.com

Library of Congress Cataloging-in-Publication Data:

Maccaro, Janet C.
  Change your food, change your mood / Janet Maccaro. -- 1st ed.
      p. cm.
  Includes bibliographical references.
  ISBN 978-1-59979-226-2
  1. Mental health--Nutritional aspects. 2. Mood (Psychology) I.
Title.

RC455.4.N8M33 2008
616.89'0654--dc22

                                    2007045911

First Edition

08 09 10 11 12 — 987654321
Printed in the United States of America

CONTENTS

PART 2: How to Feel Your Best

INTRODUCTION

IT'S TIME TO feed your brain! As the master organ of your body, your brain controls not only your intelligence and your body functions but also your emotions and moods. You cannot achieve and maintain peak function—physically, mentally, and emotionally—without the right energy-producing fuel supplied in the best amount and combination. That's why it is so important to consider what you put into your body in the form of fuel (food and supplements). What you consume affects your emotional health as much as it influences your physical and mental health. Your food really does affect your mood.

Deep within your brain is a portion known as the limbic system. In the limbic system you will find the thalamus, amygdala, hypothalamus, and more. This system deals primarily with behavior and emotions. This is the emotional storehouse of the brain where motivating feelings such as anger, fear, and pleasure are born.

Our brains become depleted just as our bodies do. So it follows that by supplementing our brains with specific nutrients, which are needed for our brains to create new neurotransmitters, we can replenish, recharge, and regenerate our brains while simultaneously focusing on nutrition to rebuild our bodies.

When I discovered this, it literally changed my life. In the past, I had been able to keep my body in balance through diet and specific supplements that were targeted to my particular areas of concern. However, this discovery about brain replenishment proved to be the missing piece of the puzzle. With this piece in place, my health—including my emotional health—could become total and complete.

I want to pass on to you what I have learned about changing the foods I eat so that I can attain and maintain healthy moods. With this knowledge comes the responsibility to share my findings, which are truly life changing.

1

HOW FOOD AFFECTS YOUR MOOD

W<small>E HAVE ALL</small> had the experience at some point—something we have eaten has had a clear and traceable effect on our emotional state. Perhaps you drank several cups of coffee along with a sugary doughnut or two. Soon afterward, you felt wired, giddy, and too jittery to complete a sentence. Some time after that, however, the bottom dropped out and your mood plummeted, along with your energy level.

What happened? All that caffeine and sugar affected you both physically and emotionally, and it was a little like being on a roller coaster. It is pure cause and effect. What you consume through your mouth, whether it is a meal, a snack, or a food supplement, can make a big difference in how you feel.

Since most of us don't particularly want to go around feeling depressed, fatigued, achy, or generally useless, it's good to learn as much as possible about how ordinary foods can enhance not only our physical state but also our emotional state. It's also good to know which foods and combinations of foods can detract from our feeling of well-being so that we can avoid them or consume them in moderation.

chapter 1

THE MIND-BODY CONNECTION

YOUR BRAIN IS responsible for all of your thought patterns, your movements, and your behaviors. It is also responsible for all of your moods and emotions, both pleasurable and painful.

CHEMICALS AND THE BRAIN

Neurotransmitters, which are important chemical messengers of the brain, help to control our feelings of anger, fear, anxiety, and depression. When neurotransmitters are depleted, prolonged anxiety or trauma can overload the cerebral cortex of the brain, causing the release of adrenaline. When adrenaline floods the brain, it triggers a multitude of life-disrupting physical symptoms.

While emotions, especially panic and anxiety, involve the brain, they are also felt throughout the entire body because our brains control every cell in the body. Biological and possibly genetic factors may be involved when people experience crippling anxiety or other emotional illnesses. It also seems that a person's perception of traumatic events or stress can actually alter his or her brain chemistry.

Emotions and the immune system

Because fear, anxiety, and other dangerous emotions can alter the brain and body's chemical balance, they have a profound influence on the development of illness. In fact, prolonged stress can lead to eventual immune system breakdown. In other words, your emotions are not just all in your head! They are linked to the chemistry of your immune system.

Candace Pert, PhD, professor at the Center for Molecular and Behavioral Neuroscience at Rutgers University, made this statement in her research on the entire physiology of the body:

> The chemical processes that mediate emotion occur not only within our brains, but also at many sites throughout the body, in fact, on the very surfaces of every single cell.[1]

Early in Dr. Pert's career she discovered a way to measure chemical receptors on cell surfaces in the brain. At this particular time, Dr. Pert was studying opiate receptors in the brain, which act like keyholes for opiate drugs such as morphine. It is the binding of an opiate to its receptor that creates the emotion of euphoria.

Soon after, it was discovered that the body makes its own opiates called *endorphins*, which serve as natural painkillers. Our bodies release these endorphins, or painkillers, during events such as childbirth and traumatic injury.

Later on, it was discovered that a host of other receptors besides opiates could be found in the brain along with other natural chemicals called neuropeptides. However, not all neuropeptides are associated with emotions as strong as euphoria. Some are more subtle, according to Dr. Pert. This groundbreaking information shocked the scientific community. The fact that endorphins were found in the immune system and that opiates and other receptors were found distributed in parts of the body outside the brain gave the mind-body connection credibility. This new research challenged the old notion that the immune system is independent of the nervous system.

Opiate receptors found in the brain were also found on immune cells. This opened the door and gave birth to mind/body medicine. Today, it is common knowledge among researchers and health-care professionals that the brain and immune system communicate with one another. Studies suggest that even very short bouts of dangerous emotions may alter some aspects of immune function.

This means that when dangerous emotions are not dealt with or when an emotionally troubling situation becomes chronic or inescapable, a person's immune system suffers and health problems

arise. In other words, people who are under stress are more suscep-
tible to illness.

The more we can learn about how our bodies react to emotional ups
and downs, the better we can cooperate with health-producing prac-
tices, including making good dietary decisions.

Moods and amino acids

How important are amino acids? Amino acids are the building
blocks of protein. Your body depends on the twenty-nine different
types of amino acids to form the sixteen hundred basic proteins
that compose 75 percent of our bodies' solid weight of structural,
muscle, and blood protein cells. Amino acids are responsible for the
growth, repair, and maintenance of your body. Most importantly,
they are sources of energy that play a vital role in the way your brain
functions.

Your brain and body cannot function without amino acids. Amino
acids heal and restore brain function because they control the anxiety
stop switch, they function as a muscle relaxant, and they act as pain
relievers. More importantly, amino acids create new neurotransmitters
for proper brain communication, helping you think better, feel better,
and stay healthy.

In her book, *The Anxiety Epidemic*, Billie Jay Sahley, PhD, states,
"There is no such thing as a tranquilizer deficiency." We may have an
amino-acid deficiency, but we in the United States definitely do not
suffer from a deficiency of prescription tranquilizers. According to
Sahley, six to ten million people in the United States alone suffer daily
from anxiety attacks, fear, panic, and phobias. Annually, these people
swallow about 982,550 pounds of medication and spend more than
$875 billion on Xanax, Zoloft, Prozac, and Valium.

If today's epidemic of anxiety, pain, stress, and emotional fatigue
can be traced to an amino-acid deficiency (rather than a tranquilizer
deficiency), this means that anything we can learn about maintaining
the healthy function of our natural amino acids through lifestyle
changes will help us replace the contents of our medicine cabinets.

KEEP A FOOD-MOOD DIARY

Writing in a diary is a good way to understand your current habits, identify areas for improvement, and recognize the progress you make.

1. Write in your journal right after you eat or finish a physical activity.
2. Be honest. Write down everything you eat, even one cookie.
3. Include drinks.
4. Write down how you are feeling. It can help you figure out if you are eating because you are hungry or for other reasons.

Review your journal at the end of each week.[2]

IDENTIFYING EMOTIONAL DISORDERS

When dangerous emotions are allowed to fester within us and we neglect to replenish our brains and bodies, full-blown emotional disorders can erupt.

The four traditional forms of treatment include behavior therapy, medication, relaxation therapy, and cognitive therapy. Most people respond best to a combination of these options.

The following disorders have become commonplace. Each one of them is caused by brain, body, and spiritual depletion, and experts agree that life events, stress, grief, anger, and heredity affect the body's internal chemistry and contribute to their development.[3]

Generalized anxiety disorder (GAD)

Anxiety and worry seem to be a normal part of our everyday lives, but excessive anxiety is more than a few butterflies in your stomach. It disrupts your life, interferes with your performance, and triggers physical discomfort. Excessive, nonspecific anxiety can be labeled generalized anxiety disorder, or GAD for short.

GAD is marked by excessive and unrealistic worries about health, money, or career prospects that last for six months or longer. Keep in mind that realistic anxiety, such as financial concerns after losing a job, is to be expected. However, if you worry excessively over events that are unlikely to occur, you may be struggling with GAD. People who live with GAD typically have a number of physical and emotional complaints, including insomnia, dizziness, concentration problems, sore muscles, restlessness, and irritability. Symptoms can vary from person to person, but at least six of these indicators must be present for a diagnosis of GAD.

More than five out of every one hundred people will develop GAD at some point in their lives. Researchers have not identified a cause for GAD, but biological factors, life experiences, and family background all appear to play a part. The disorder tends to occur starting in the early twenties, but it can also begin in childhood. Others report having their first battle with GAD after the age of thirty.

Too much stress often triggers this disorder. In the months or years immediately prior to the onset of GAD, many sufferers report an increase in stressful life events, such as illness, job loss, death in the family, or divorce. Positive life events can also be stressful. Happy occasions, such as marriage, a new baby, or a new career, can also be catalysts for the development of GAD.

While medications can be extremely helpful in the treatment of GAD, other helpful strategies include exercising for thirty minutes daily, receiving a massage, prayer, and controlled breathing. Some of the supplements discussed later in this book will also help to replenish the brain and body, including GABA (gamma-aminobutyric acid), magnesium, and the full spectrum of amino acids. My progressive muscle relaxation technique, MANTLE, has also helped many GAD sufferers.

What is it? It's very simple. My MANTLE technique involves simply tensing and holding for the count of ten each part of your body, one section at a time. To remind myself that I need attention daily, I coined the acronym MANTLE:

M—Muscles

A—Always

N—Need

T—Tension

L—Loosening

E—Every day

Begin with your eyes; tense and hold them shut for ten seconds, then release. Take a deep, cleansing breath. (Try to breathe from your belly; fill your lungs and raise your diaphragm and then exhale slowly through your mouth.) Next, tighten all of the muscles of your face and mouth, make a face, and hold it for ten seconds. Relax and take another deep, cleansing breath. Continue this tensing and releasing exercise on down through the other parts of your body: shoulders, arms, hands, fingers, upper abdomen, lower abdomen and pelvic area, upper thighs, calves, feet, toes.

Although anxiety is among the most common, most treatable mental disorders, relief from GAD does not happen overnight. It will take some time and dedication to achieve lasting results.

Social anxiety disorder

This is more than just a case of being shy. Shy people may be extremely self-conscious, but they do not experience avoidance behavior, physical symptoms, and crippling feelings known as anticipatory anxiety.

Social phobia is an anxiety disorder that tends to begin in the mid to late teen years and can grow worse over time. The central fear in this disorder is embarrassment over the way one might act while performing a task in public. An example would be public speaking, which is the most common form of a social phobia. Others include the fear of parties or celebrations, eating in restaurants, flying in a full plane, or riding in a bus or car.

Social phobics are acutely aware of physical signs of nervousness such as trembling, blushing, and sweating. Sufferers feel so much extreme anxiety over upcoming public encounters that their nervousness can create the poor performance they're afraid of. This only intensifies future worry. Researchers believe that this disorder is caused by biological or genetic factors along with experiences such as a publicly embarrassing or humiliating experience at an impressionable age.

Thirteen out of every one hundred Americans have a chance of developing this disorder at some point in their lives. Phobias can disrupt family life, limit productivity, reduce self-esteem, and break the spirit. The standard treatments for this disorder include medications, behavior therapy, relaxation techniques, and cognitive therapy. Training in social skills is of additional benefit.

Obsessive-compulsive disorder (OCD)

"Lather, rinse, repeat." A person with OCD may feel they must perform a ritual such as this over and over. Some sufferers spend hours bathing, shampooing, washing their hands, or cleaning their homes. Although they perform such routines in an effort to relieve their extreme anxiety, these ritualistic behaviors interfere with the person's daily activities.

People with OCD have a fear of uncertainty and constant doubts. They seek much reassurance from others. Many people with OCD also suffer from depression. This can be a very tiring disorder.

Evidence suggests that biological factors play a part in the development of OCD, and there is an observable tendency for it to run in families. Experts believe that OCD is a neurobiological illness that is influenced by life events. It does respond to treatment, and help is available. If you suffer from OCD, don't hide your condition from others—seek help.

You may see your physician or therapist for medication tailored to your needs. Your nutritional depletion must also be addressed. GABA and B vitamins can be of help. When your brain is restored, your emotional issues can be resolved.

WHAT ARE THE SYMPTOMS OF OCD?
People with OCD:

Have repeated thoughts or images about many different things, such as fear of germs, dirt, or intruders; violence; hurting loved ones; sexual acts; conflicts with religious beliefs; or being overly neat.

Do the same rituals over and over such as washing hands, locking and unlocking doors, counting, keeping unneeded items, or repeating the same steps again and again.

Have unwanted thoughts and behaviors they can't control.

Don't get pleasure from the behaviors or rituals but get brief relief from the anxiety the thoughts cause.

Spend at least an hour a day on thoughts and rituals, which cause distress and get in the way of daily life.[4]

Post-traumatic stress disorder (PTSD)

With PTSD, your past literally comes back to haunt you. In the past, it was called "combat fatigue" and was thought to affect only soldiers and veterans. Now we know that this disorder affects anyone, male or female.

All of us look backward at times. Thinking about happy moments from our past makes us feel good, but other memories have the opposite effect. When death or some other personal tragedy happens, we may mourn and undergo difficulties for a period of time, but eventually we put the past aside and get on with our lives. For some people, however, this is impossible. They are affected so profoundly by their experiences that they cannot live a normal life.

PTSD is characterized by irritability, nightmares, flashbacks, and feeling the need to be constantly vigilant. As it becomes a chronic problem, brain depletion occurs. Ongoing stress can make changes even in the structure of the brain. In addition, high blood pressure, cancer, and heart disease have been associated with this condition if it is left untreated.

The events most likely to trigger this disorder are the unexpected death of a loved one, being assaulted, or being raped. Other triggers include auto accidents, a cancer diagnosis, miscarriage, and traumatic childbirth. These are experiences that happen to large numbers of Americans.

The most common symptoms of PTSD are flashbacks, fear, and insomnia. Other troubling symptoms include "jumping out of your skin" when someone enters a room and avoiding people, places, smells, and clothes that remind a person of a traumatic event. In some cases, people avoid intimacy because they simply cannot get close to anyone sexually. PTSD sufferers keep a wall up between themselves and the world. If PTSD symptoms linger for more than a month, chances are they will become chronic.

If you think you are suffering from PTSD, what do you do? Where do you start?

Begin by talking. The best thing you can do after any traumatic event is talk about it. At the same time, feed your brain amino acids such as GABA to help create new neurotransmitters. I recommend a yeast-, sugar-, and dairy-free eating plan. Focus on your adrenal health (see "Addressing Adrenal Exhaustion" in chapter 3). For additional help, visit the Web site of the Anxiety Disorders Association of America (ADAA) at www.adaa.org.

RECOGNIZING POST-TRAUMATIC STRESS DISORDER

Have you lived through a scary and dangerous event? Please put a check in the box next to any problems you have:

- ❏ Sometimes, all of a sudden, I feel like the event is happening again. I never know when this will occur.
- ❏ I have nightmares and bad memories of the terrifying event.
- ❏ I stay away from places that remind me of the event.
- ❏ I jump and feel very upset when something happens without warning.
- ❏ I have a hard time trusting or feeling close to other people.
- ❏ I get mad very easily.
- ❏ I feel guilty because others died and I lived.
- ❏ I have trouble sleeping, and my muscles are tense.[5]

Panic disorder

Nearly three million adult Americans will suffer from a panic disorder at some point in their lives. These numbers are scary enough to make anyone panic!

Panic disorder is highly treatable once it is diagnosed. This disorder appears to run in families and is two to three times more likely to strike women. As with other anxiety disorders, the first attack is often preceded by a stressful event such as the death of a parent, a move to a new city, or the breakup of a marriage.

With panic disorder, you may need medication initially to stop the attacks. Over the long term, GABA (gamma-aminobutyric acid) and the full spectrum of amino acids, along with dietary changes, emotional release techniques, and spiritual growth, will ensure positive results.

DO YOU HAVE PANIC DISORDER?

Do you have sudden bursts of fear for no reason? Do you feel awful when they happen? Please put a check in the box next to any problems you have during these sudden bursts of fear.

❑ I have chest pains or a racing heart.

❑ I have a hard time breathing.

❑ I have a choking feeling.

❑ I feel dizzy.

❑ I sweat a lot.

❑ I have stomach problems or feel like I need to throw up.

❑ I shake, tremble, or tingle.

❑ I feel out of control.

❑ I feel unreal.

❑ I am afraid I am dying or going crazy.

If you put a check in the box next to some of these problems, you may have panic disorder.[6]

THE MEDICATION MAZE

Most anxiety disorders have a biological component and therefore respond to medication. These medications can be used over the short term, or they may be required for a lengthy period of time. With medication, anxiety symptoms are reduced, and it is easier for a person, alone or with a therapist, to find and address the root cause of his or her emotional distress. If underlying causes, including brain depletion, are not addressed, a person ends up becoming one of the millions of Americans who need to stay on medication just to function day to day.

The following types of medications are routinely prescribed to help with the symptoms of anxiety disorders:

1. *Selective serotonin reuptake inhibitors (SSRIs)* are considered a first line of treatment for panic disorder, social phobia, OCD, PTSD, and GAD. Traditionally, they have been used to treat depression. They need to be taken only once a day, and they have become among the most widely used drugs in the world. Common side effects are

mild nausea and sexual dysfunction, which may resolve over time.

2. *Monoamine oxidase (MAO) inhibitors* are powerful drugs used in the treatment of panic disorder, social phobia, PTSD, and OCD. Some doctors prefer to try other treatments first, in part because MAO inhibitors require the patient to restrict alcohol consumption, other medications, and certain foods, including cheeses that contain tyramine.

3. *Tricyclics (TCAs),* first created for treating depression, are also effective in blocking panic attacks. They reduce symptoms of PTSD and can be effective against OCD. Tricyclics take two to three weeks to take effect. Their most bothersome side effect is weight gain, followed by drowsiness, dizziness, dry mouth, and impaired sexual function.

4. *Beta blockers* are often prescribed for those with social phobia. These drugs reduce anxiety symptoms such as heart palpitations, sweating, and tremors, and they can control anxiety in public situations. Beta blockers reduce blood pressure and slow the heartbeat.

5. *Benzodiazepines* are effective against GAD. Some drugs in this category are also used to treat panic disorder and social phobia. They are relatively fast acting. The most common side effect is drowsiness; they also have a potential for dependency. Anxiety symptoms, as well as withdrawal symptoms, may return when the drug is discontinued.

6. *Anticonvulsants,* primarily designed to prevent or stop seizures, can sometimes be used to treat social phobia.

Brain Food for Your Mood

Since both emotional disorders and physical disorders are mind/body connected, they aggravate and intensify each other because of the close relationship between your brain and your body. Sometimes it seems like the more you struggle to rise above your disorders and difficulties, the worse it gets. Your extremely tensed state interferes with proper sleep and eventually leads to fatigue and emotional despair or breakdown.

With your brain becoming as depleted as your body, it follows that by supplementing our brains with specific nutrients that are needed for our brains to create new neurotransmitters, we can refresh and renew our brains while simultaneously focusing on nutrition to rebuild our bodies.

As you move into the next chapter and keep reading, you will discover how you can choose the best "brain foods" for your mood.

BRAIN FOODS FOR YOUR MOOD

Choose to:

Drink more water
Eat more fresh fruits and vegetables
Eat more fish
Eat more "brown" (whole-grain) foods
Eat more protein
Eat more nuts and seeds
Eat more fiber and more organic food

Cut back on:

Sugar
Caffeine
Alcohol
Saturated fats
Food that contains additives
Dairy and/or wheat products[7]

chapter 2

HORMONES AND YOUR DIET

FROM THE CRADLE to the grave, a woman's hormones play a vitally important role in her health and well-being—so much so that hundreds of books have been written on the topic.

Today's women are not sitting back and letting symptoms of hormonal imbalance or depletion destroy their lives, health, and peace of mind. Our mothers and grandmothers were not as fortunate, but for the most part, their hormonal issues were not as severe as the ones we face in this era. This is due in part to the amount of environmental and dietary xenoestrogens to which we are exposed on a daily basis. *Xenoestrogens* are substances that exert an estrogen-like effect on our systems, thereby contributing to hormonal imbalance due to estrogen dominance. It is this estrogen dominance that causes early puberty in young girls. When you add in lowered adrenal function (hypoadrenalism) and sugar consumption, you have the makings of a nation of hormonally imbalanced women.

The good news is that whatever the hormonal stage a woman is in—PMS, perimenopause, or menopause—there are answers from nature that can help bring balance back.

PMS: THE PERIOD BEFORE YOUR PERIOD

It has been observed that 90 percent of premenopausal women suffer from some degree of premenstrual syndrome (PMS). The symptoms—which include mood swings, headaches, acne, bloating, irritability, fatigue, tender breasts, anxiety, depression, low back pain, and more—can last from two days to as long as two weeks and are caused by the hormonal shift in estrogen and progesterone levels during the menstrual cycle.

In brief, PMS results from inadequate levels of progesterone in the second half of the menstrual cycle. This creates an "estrogen dominant" situation. Estrogen dominance occurs more often because of xenoestrogens such as environmental pollutants, pesticides, plastic-lined cans, stress, and foods (in particular, beef, poultry, and milk) laden with growth hormones. In addition, a diet that contains too much salt, caffeine, sugar, and red meat are all implicated in the development of PMS. It has been found that many PMS sufferers also have deficiencies in the B vitamins and in minerals.

The following recommendations will provide your body with nutrition and supplemental support necessary for relief of symptoms of PMS. These recommendations may take two or three full monthly cycles to take full effect. You will need to be consistent in applying the changes to your diet in order to maintain your improvement.

PMS diet protocol

Your diet should be low in fat and should include regular seafood consumption. Be sure to eat plenty of cruciferous vegetables (broccoli, cauliflower) and dark, leafy greens to reduce estrogen buildup. Prepare brown rice often to obtain B vitamins.

Buy organic meats, milk, milk products, and canned foods. Eliminate dairy products completely during your premenstrual days.

Use whole grains, and keep your diet low in sugar and salt. Avoid caffeine and animal products as much as possible.

HOW TO GET MORE FIBER IN YOUR DIET

To get more fiber in your diet naturally, choose foods that are high in fiber, such as:

- Beans and legumes, cooked from dry or canned—navy beans, kidney beans, black beans, pinto beans, lima beans, white beans, great northern beans, soybeans, split peas, lentils, chickpeas
- Fresh fruits and vegetables, with skins/peels when possible—prunes, artichokes, sweet potatoes, green peas, pears, apples, bananas, oranges, parsnips, potatoes
- Whole grains such as bulgar or barley, whole-grain pastas and whole-grain breads (wheat, millet, rye, etc.)
- Nuts, especially almonds
- Raw bran or oat bran cereals and baked products

To keep your bowel function optimal, add fiber to your diet and drink plenty of water. To help control premenstrual cravings for sweets (mainly chocolate and refined sugar), increased appetite, headaches, and fatigue, consider the following supplements:

- Balanced B-complex vitamin: 50–100 mg of each B vitamin
- Chromium picolinate: 200 mcg daily (400 mcg if over 150 pounds)
- Calcium: 800–1,200 mg daily
- Magnesium: 400–800 mg daily

In addition, split your daily meals into many small meals, taken throughout the day.

To balance your estrogen/progesterone ratio, use a natural progesterone cream applied topically twice daily for two weeks prior to the expected beginning of your menstrual period. Your mineral intake will be boosted if you take calcium and magnesium in the dosages indicated above.

To ease your water retentiveness (which is why you have breast tenderness, bloating, and headaches), eliminate caffeine and chocolate.

You can also use evening primrose oil (3,000 mg daily) and ginkgo biloba. To relieve lower back pain, take quercetin (1,000 mg) or bromelain (1,500 mg), or use ginger packs.

COMMON FOOD SOURCES OF QUERCETIN[1]

Apple skin (raw)	Cocoa powder, dry
Argula (raw)	Cranberries
Asparagus (raw)	Elderberries
Black currants	Fennel leaves
Black grapes	Green beans
Black plums (raw)	Green tea (brewed)
Black tea (brewed)	Hot peppers (raw)
Blackberries	Kale
Blueberries	Lettuce
Broccoli (raw)	Mulberries
Broccoli raab (Rapini)	Onions
Buckwheat	Pear skin (raw)
Capers	Purple plums (raw)
Carob flour	Raspberries
Cherries	Red grapes
Cherry tomatoes	Yellow snap beans
Chicory greens (raw)	

AFTER THE FALL:
CRAVINGS, CALORIES, AND HORMONES

Perimenopause occurs in women around the age of forty and continues until the early fifties when the menstrual period becomes a thing of the past, signaling the beginning of menopause. During this stage of life, many women experience a decrease or even a cessation in their progesterone production because of irregular ovarian cycling and ovarian aging. At the same time, estrogen levels may be excessively or moderately high, causing a troubling, continual state of imbalance.

Women may experience a plethora of symptoms, some for years on end. These may include mood swings, fatigue, breast tenderness, foggy thinking, irritability, headaches, insomnia, decreased sex drive, anxiety, depression, allergy symptoms (including asthma), fat gain (especially around the middle), hair loss, memory loss, water retention, bone loss, slow metabolism, endometrial and breast cancers, and many more. In other words, hormonal imbalance has far-reaching effects on many tissues in the body, including the heart, brain, blood vessels, bones, uterus, and breasts.

The key to smooth perimenopause is bringing the levels of estrogen and progesterone back into balance as well as managing stress. To bring the hormone levels back into balance, I recommend using natural progesterone. According to the late pioneer of progesterone therapy, John R. Lee, MD, "One of progesterone's most powerful and important roles in the body is to balance and oppose estrogen."[2] Natural progesterone has been found to be effective in combating perimenopausal anxiety and mood swings. In addition, it plays a very important part in the prevention and reversal of osteoporosis. Natural progesterone offers a woman all of these benefits without hormone replacement therapy (HRT). The recommended dosage for women in perimenopause is ¼ to ½ teaspoon applied to any clean area of skin twice a day (morning and evening).

If you do your best to maintain your physical, mental, and emotional balance through the middle season of your life, the process of aging will be more graceful and less painful for you.

Natural supplements

There are natural supplements that you can use to deal with any of the perimenopausal symptoms you are experiencing. Try the following perimenopausal marvels in your daily regimen:

- *Quercetin* is a potent antioxidant that reduces the inflammation of endometriosis. It also helps reduce estrogen and cholesterol levels while boosting circulation and proper digestion.

- *Chaste tree berry* promotes progesterone production.

- *Bromelain* is a digestive enzyme that reduces pain and inflammation when taken between meals.

- *Flaxseed oil* will help you increase your intake of *essential fatty acids*, which will help to reduce pain due to bloating, breast tenderness, endometriosis, and menstrual cramping. Essential fatty acids are also good for skin, hair, and the heart.

- *Vitamin C* has additional wide-reaching benefits.

FOOD SOURCES OF VITAMIN C[3]

Food, Standard Amount	Vitamin C (mg)	Calories
Guava, raw, ½ cup	188	56
Red sweet pepper, raw, ½ cup	142	20
Red sweet pepper, cooked, ½ cup	116	19
Kiwi fruit, 1 medium	70	46
Orange, raw, 1 medium	70	62
Orange juice, ¾ cup	61–93	79–84
Green pepper, sweet, raw, ½ cup	60	15
Green pepper, sweet, cooked, ½ cup	51	19
Grapefruit juice, ¾ cup	50–70	71–86
Vegetable juice cocktail, ¾ cup	50	34
Strawberries, raw, ½ cup	49	27
Brussels sprouts, cooked, ½ cup	48	28
Cantaloupe, ¼ medium	47	51
Papaya, raw, ¼ medium	47	30
Kohlrabi, cooked, ½ cup	45	24
Broccoli, raw, ½ cup	39	15
Edible pod peas, cooked, ½ cup	38	34
Broccoli, cooked, ½ cup	37	26
Sweet potato, canned, ½ cup	34	116

FOOD SOURCES OF VITAMIN C[3]

Food, Standard Amount	Vitamin C (mg)	Calories
Tomato juice, ¾ cup	33	31
Cauliflower, cooked, ½ cup	28	17
Pineapple, raw, ½ cup	28	37
Kale, cooked, ½ cup	27	18
Mango, ½ cup	23	54

On to menopause

It is unfortunate that many in the medical profession have tended to treat this phase of life as a disease state rather than as a normal passage of life. In years past, women with these symptoms (see chart on next page) were nurtured with herbs, reassurance, and time-tested wisdom from older women who had taken the journey before them. With today's hectic lifestyle and relentlessly high stress levels, hormone levels fall down even farther.

Menopause can vary widely between individuals. Many factors influence the timing of menopause, including trauma, surgery, and low body weight (which brings on early menopause due to decreased hormone output by the ovaries). Anorexia can cause the ovaries to shut down completely. Conversely, being overweight can delay menopause because extra fat increases estradiol in a woman's body. Physically active and well-nourished women experience late menopause while smokers experience earlier menopause. Adrenal exhaustion from too much stress and poor diet can cause early menopause.

MENOPAUSE

Do you have any of these symptoms?

- ❏ Irregular periods
- ❏ Weight gain
- ❏ Diagnosed with uterine fibroids
- ❏ Sore and lumpy breasts
- ❏ Drier, thinner, and more wrinkled skin, lacking that velvety texture
- ❏ Decreased sex drive, painful intercourse
- ❏ Irritability, anxiety, and maybe even depression
- ❏ Frequent bladder or vaginal infections
- ❏ Achy joints and muscles
- ❏ Forgetfulness
- ❏ Hot flashes and "electric shocks" going through your body
- ❏ Insomnia

Welcome to your menopausal years, the transitional midlife stage!

What is a hot flash anyway? Hot flashes are related to fluctuating estrogen levels. They occur as a result of increased blood flow to the brain, skin, and internal organs, which causes a sudden sensation of warmth, sometimes followed by a deep sense of being chilled. At menopause, estrogen production drops by 75–90 percent, while progesterone production virtually stops. Androgens, the hormones that stimulate your sex drive, drop by 50 percent.

HORMONES FROM PLANTS IN YOUR DIET

Midlife women today are at a crossroad. Do they take estrogen and risk hormone-related cancer later on, or do they suffer in silence as their bodies ache and rapidly age? Do they live in a hormone-deficient state and subject themselves to the possibility of acquiring the degenerative diseases that attack a body lacking proper balance? Or do they seek a natural transition?

Let's talk about why a natural transition is best. It is common knowledge that the risks associated with conventional HRT have filled medical journals for more than twenty years. The good news is that you do not have to suffer with the symptoms of accelerated aging and degenerative health conditions that often result from conventional HRT therapy. There are many natural supplements that can be just as effective—or more effective—for dealing with the onset of menopause.

Bioidentical hormone replacement therapy

In our younger days, our bodies made ample hormones to keep us young, healthy, and vibrant. As the years pass, our bodies do not produce hormones in the balanced amounts that keep us feeling energized. What can we do? The answer is simple. We can turn to the plant kingdom, where natural hormones abound. Soybeans, black cohosh, Mexican wild yam, and licorice can be of benefit to a perimenopausal/menopausal woman. For many women, stressful lifestyles have made it necessary to move up to bioidentical hormones that are derived from these plants and then synthesized in a lab to be molecularly similar to the hormones our bodies make—estrogen, progesterone, DHEA, and so forth. This is unlike synthetic hormones, which the drug companies purposely make different in order to patent the drugs such as Prempro, Provera, and Premarin.

Bioidentical hormones are much safer for your body because they are easier for your body to metabolize without many of the side effects that synthetic hormones create. They have been shown to increase your energy, improve your sense of well-being, improve your memory, aid weight loss, increase libido, and reduce facial hair. Conversely, synthetic hormones have side effects that include lack of sex drive, poor sleep, increased cancer risk, and weight gain.

Neither bioidentical hormones nor synthetic hormones can do the whole job alone. You must clean up your diet, eat sensibly and often, get plenty of rest, drink plenty of water, and take a calcium supplement and a good daily multivitamin, taking particular concern for the health of your adrenal glands because they play an important role in your hormone balance.

MENOPAUSE DIETARY GUIDELINES

You should follow these dietary guidelines to help ease the symptoms of menopause:

- Add soy foods to your diet.
- Limit sugar, sodium, caffeine, pies, cakes, and pastries.
- Limit red meat.
- Eat fresh vegetables, fruits, and nuts.
- Instead of three large meals a day, eat several smaller meals throughout the day.
- Limit dairy products.

In addition to dietary changes, be sure to make some important lifestyle changes that bring you a daily dose of exercise, laughter, and relaxation (which can include deep breathing and massage).

WATCH YOUR SODIUM

In the typical American diet, the relative amounts of dietary sodium come from the following sources:[4]

Food processing—77 percent

Naturally occurring—12 percent

At the table—6 percent

During cooking—5 percent

To watch your sodium intake, pay close attention to the nutrition labels on foods and beverages that you buy in the grocery store, and be careful what you choose when you eat away from home.

There are also many natural herbal remedies that can alleviate your menopause symptoms and help you find balance in this season of life. I suggest that you try them one by one and determine for yourself the ones that really give you comfort:

- 5-HTP (5-hydroxytryptophan, for insomnia and anxiety at night)

- Bioflavonoids (also high in phytoestrogens)
- Black cohosh
- Black currant seed oil
- Dong quai (high in phytoestrogens)
- Licorice (for your adrenal health)
- Plant enzymes (taken with meals)
- Red raspberry
- Vitamin B-complex
- Vitamin C
- Vitamin E (normalizes hormones)

Menopause does not signal the end of your vitality, attractiveness, and purpose in life. It is a time of reevaluation and a time to focus on the rest of your life and accomplishing the desires of your heart. It is a time for wisdom gained and shared. It is a wonderful time of service, self-discovery, and spiritual maturity. Many women experience "post-menopausal zest" for life. May you be one of them!

RECOMMENDED EATING PLAN FOR MENOPAUSE[5]

- Boost your daily intake of fruits. Choose melons, bananas, and citrus fruits like oranges and lemons, which are high in potassium. Potassium-rich foods help balance sodium and water retention. Also include some dried fruit like apricots and figs.

- Boost your daily intake of vegetables (including salads). In particular, choose yams, dark leafy vegetables such as kale, collard greens, spinach, pak choi, broccoli, and cabbage, as well as peppers, tomatoes, and a variety of others.

- Introduce soy foods into your daily diet. Choose soybeans and foods made from soybeans, such as calcium-fortified soy milk, soy yogurt, and tofu.

- Eat regular amounts of fiber.

- Stop frying your foods; instead, broil or bake them.

- Get rid of white bread and products made from white flour. Choose whole-grain breads, oats, rye, wheat germ, etc.

- Eliminate white rice (except basmati), and switch to long-grain brown rice.

- Eat fewer regular white potatoes and more sweet potatoes and pasta.

- Add regular helpings of beans and lentils to your meals.

- Replace processed cooking oils with unprocessed oils. Choose extra-virgin olive oil, canola, and flaxseed oil.

- Make oily fish (salmon, mackerel) a regular feature of your diet. Oily fish is rich in omega-3 essential fatty acids, which provide a huge range of health benefits.

- Try adding seaweed to your diet; ask at your local health food store. Choose Nori, Wakame, Kombu, Arame, which contain natural hormones and plant chemicals to help you during menopause.

- Drink more mineral/bottled water, less caffeine, and little to no alcohol.

- Enjoy high-calorie junk foods as an occasional treat only.

chapter 3

STRESS AND YOUR DIET

T O ONE DEGREE or another, all of us experience stress on a daily basis. Some of it, especially if it is cumulative, can set us up for an instinctive "fight-or-flight" response.

Exactly what happens to you when you experience extreme stress? The rate of your breathing increases to supply the necessary oxygen to your heart. Your heart rate increases to force more blood to your muscles and brain. Your liver dumps more stored glucose into your bloodstream to energize your body so that it can support an increased level of physical activity. You produce more sweat to eliminate toxic compounds produced by your body and to lower your body temperature.

Stress contributes greatly to the development of most disorders. Stress is a component in everything from generalized anxiety to fibromyalgia, and improvement will be slower unless it is addressed.

Do you suffer from troublesome maladies? Remember, your current state of health developed over many years. The good news is that even though you may feel defeated, you still have a level of good health, and you can build on it.

HOW STRESS AFFECTS YOUR BODY

Stress builds up over time, and different types of stressors affect people in different ways. What does your own body reveal about the level of stress you may be undergoing?

Low-level stress can manifest itself in subtle ways, such as short-temperedness, scowling or frowning, having "tired eyes," exhibiting a bored or a nervous demeanor, or losing interest in activities that used to be enjoyable.

If this level of stress is not addressed over time, another layer of stress gets added on top of it that includes increased fatigue, insomnia, overall sadness, outbursts of anger, fear, and even paranoia.

On top of that level of stress, underlying physical problems may begin to emerge, such as chronic head and neck pain, high blood pressure, an upset stomach, and an overall aged appearance.

People who are even more stressed develop frequent infections and illnesses. In chapter 1 we talked about how stress can reduce a person's immunity and resistance. Stress-related ailments can include skin disorders, asthma, heart disease, kidney malfunction, and mental/emotional breakdown.

Learn to recognize the early signs of stress, and take action as soon as possible to combat it through exercise, relaxation, dietary changes, and prayer.

Learning to relax is one of the most crucial components of reducing the effects of stress. Obviously, it is far more desirable to live in a relaxed state in which your body and brain are not working overtime. By implementing the lifestyle changes you will find in this book, you can learn how to relax.

In summary, here is what you want to achieve:

- Reduced heart rate and blood pressure
- Decreased rate of breathing
- Improved digestion
- Lower blood sugar levels

Don't let stress become a destructive force that robs you of your quality of life and well-being.

How Stress Affects Your Brain

Emotional fatigue is another manifestation of stress. When you have reacted repeatedly in an emotional way (anger, impatience, tears, or any emotion, even excitement), it's not uncommon to feel drained or as if your batteries are dead. In a sense, it's true.

Your adrenal glands are the two little glands that sit on top of each kidney. I call them your *A batteries*. Your adrenal glands help your body deal with stress. They secrete adrenaline in crisis situations to give you the extra energy you need to handle an immediate crisis. They are part of your "fight-or-flight" response.

In days gone by, the fight-or-flight response was useful. It still is, once in a while, to get us out of the way of an oncoming automobile or the like, but when we get stuck in emergency mode because of our stressful lifestyles, our brains tell our adrenal glands to provide a steady stream of adrenaline, which was never intended. Not only do our adrenal glands get exhausted, but we do too. Handicapped, our poor brains struggle to supply the right information at the right time. We make bad decisions, fall under the influence of rogue emotional responses, and generally do poorly.

When our A batteries are drained we feel sluggish and lethargic; our memories are dull; we get moody and touchy; and we feel anxious, weak, and shaky. We may also suffer from hypoglycemia, low immunity, dry skin, brittle nails, sugar cravings, and profound fatigue.

CHECK YOUR BATTERIES

If you want to see just how well your adrenal glands are performing, try this self-test. First, lie down and rest for five minutes. Then take your blood pressure. Stand up immediately and take your blood pressure reading once more.

If your blood pressure is lower after you stand up, you probably have reduced adrenal gland function, which means your batteries need a charge. The lower the blood pressure reading is from your resting blood pressure, the more severe your low adrenal function is.

The systolic number (the number on top of the blood pressure reading) normally is about ten points higher when you are standing than when you lie down. A difference of more than ten points should be addressed.

There's help. Pay attention to your adrenal glands, your vital "batteries," as you work to restore your system after a time of grief or conflict, prolonged pain syndromes, anxiety disorders, or depression.

ADDRESSING ADRENAL EXHAUSTION—DIET AND LIFESTYLE

When your adrenal glands are in trouble, you must address lifestyle habits that are destroying them. By this I mean you make sure you are eating healthy foods (which will mean eliminating caffeine and sugar) and are getting enough sleep daily.

Hippocrates said, "Let food be your medicine and medicine be your food."

Your diet should contain seafood, brown rice, and green "super foods" such as Kyo-Green (available at your local health-food store), which contain protein and all the B vitamins.

Exercise is another way to boost your adrenal health because it releases stress and tension. Just don't overdo it. In moderation, regular exercise will help diffuse and release your daily stress.

Sleep is crucial. During the night your body has a chance to heal and regenerate. Your nervous system gets a break from the devastating effects of dangerous emotions. Sleep recharges not only the adrenal glands but also your entire system.

An adrenal glandular supplement will help to nourish and stimulate your exhausted adrenals. It will also help to reduce inflammation and increase body tone and endurance that is so often lost when we are depleted. When vitamins B and C are added or included in the adrenal glandular supplement, the results are even better. Candida, chronic fatigue syndrome, allergies, and blood sugar imbalances such as hypoglycemia and diabetes are greatly improved by taking an adrenal glandular supplement.

Your adrenal exhaustion may have been caused by unrelenting stress, or it may have come from long-term use of corticosteroid drugs for asthma, arthritis, or allergies. Too much sugar and caffeine in your diet or deficiencies of vitamins B and C can also contribute to adrenal exhaustion. Adrenal exhaustion is also common during the perimenopausal and menopausal stage of a woman's life.

So, if you are suffering from several of the symptoms on the following list, you can jump-start your A batteries again by trying the protocol you will see after the list.

Symptoms

- ❑ Severe reactions to odors or certain foods
- ❑ Recurring yeast infections
- ❑ Heart palpitations and panic attacks
- ❑ Dry skin and peeling nails
- ❑ Clammy hands and soles of feet
- ❑ Low energy and poor memory
- ❑ Chronic lower-back pain
- ❑ Cravings for salt and sugar

Protocols

1. Rest, rest, rest!
2. Get regular exercise in moderation.
3. Add the following to your daily supplements: vitamin C and B-complex, pantothenic acid, tyrosine (an amino acid).
4. Use an adrenal glandular supplement, which you can find at your local health food store.
5. Add foods to your diet that will support good adrenal health. These include brown rice, almonds, garlic, salmon, flounder, lentils, sunflower seeds, bran, brewers yeast, and avocados.
6. Begin to use two teaspoonfuls of royal jelly daily. This substance is the food of queen bees, and it is marketed in health-food stores. It is rich in vitamins, minerals, enzymes, and hormones, and it possesses antibiotic and antibacterial properties as well as a high concentration of pantothenic acid.

AN ANTISTRESS DIET

If you are feeling stressed, try this menu plan:

Breakfast:	Make a smoothie using a banana, several large chunks of pineapple, and the juice of a large orange.
Midmorning snack:	Munch on lightly toasted walnuts and dried dates. Instead of caffeinated tea or coffee, which can just fuel your stress levels, try an herbal tea.
Lunch:	Make a fresh pasta salad the night before, and store it in a plastic container. While the pasta is still warm, drizzle it with a light lemon vinaigrette made with fresh lemon juice, olive oil, sea salt, and black pepper. Fold in a small can of tuna, a handful of baby spinach leaves, and half a diced sweet red pepper.
Dinner:	Stress depletes the body of vitamin C, and both sweet and new potatoes are excellent sources of this essential vitamin. Wash four or five small sweet potatoes and one regular size white potato and cut into bite-sized chunks. Drizzle with a little olive oil, sea salt, and pepper and roast in the oven for forty-five to fifty minutes. Wrap a piece of fresh fish in aluminum foil with a few slices of lemon and scatter with sprigs of fresh parsley or thyme. Place in the oven fifteen minutes before the potatoes are done. Oily fish such as salmon, mackerel, and tuna contain polyunsaturated omega-3 fatty acids. Serve with some steamed broccoli—another vegetable high in vitamin C—sprinkled with sesame seeds, which provide calcium.[1]

Refer to chapter 5, "Depression and Your Diet" for more information about amino acids as natural tranquilizers.

chapter 4

FATIGUE AND YOUR DIET

THERE'S SUCH A difference between being simply tired and being truly fatigued. You can become tired from a restless night or the physical exertion of jogging or a long and demanding day at your job. After a relaxing weekend, you feel fine again. You don't keep thinking, "I'm so tired."

But when day after day you wake up in the morning tired, you feel like your brain is in a cloud all day long, the idea of a nap suggests itself regularly, and you can't stop thinking, "I'm so tired," you are probably suffering from fatigue.

You can address fatigue in practical ways, and you should start with that. Are you making an effort to get enough sleep? Are you overcommitting yourself to activities and stretching yourself to the limit of your daily endurance? Perhaps you can make some changes in your lifestyle.

In the meantime, and along with other changes in your life, how can you address fatigue nutritionally?

TAKE A LOOK AT SUGAR

Do you reach for sugar in times of stress, depression, or anxiety? Sugar is especially detrimental to your brain and body function. Excessive sugar also suppresses your body's immune response. If you are consuming too much sugar on a daily basis, you may be setting yourself up for low blood sugar. Many people who suffer from anxiety and depression also have to deal with hypoglycemia. Notice how the symptoms of anxiety are identical to the following profile of a hypoglycemic individual—and how fatigue is at the head of the list:

- Fatigue
- Rapid pulse
- Heart palpitations
- Cold sweats
- Twitching
- Crying spells
- Weakness
- Irritability
- Nightmares
- Poor concentration

If these symptoms are familiar to you, you must focus on eating more fiber and protein at each meal and cutting back on simple sugar. It is very important for you to have a high-protein snack between meals. This will keep your blood sugar levels stable all day long.

FOODS HIGH IN SUGAR

To control your sugar intake, watch out for the following foods:

All sweet desserts and snacks

All non-diet sodas and fruit drinks with added sugar

All foods processed with added sugar (watch for "sugars" on the nutritional label)

Dried fruits such as raisins, frozen or canned fruits packed in sugar syrup

Sweetened, flavored milk products

Limiting (and especially eliminating) sugar will not be easy to achieve, but for you to rebuild your brain and body, your sugar consumption *must* be curtailed. The following dietary guidelines can help you make the adjustment:

- Chromium picolinate
- B-complex vitamins
- Vitamin C
- Pantothenic acid
- Adrenal gland supplement

- Calcium and magnesium
- A protein shake each morning
- Stevia extract used instead of sugar as a sweetener
- Fiber (brown rice, for example)

It would be wise for you to work to balance your blood sugar now, because low blood sugar can predispose you to develop diabetes later in your life. Diabetes occurs when the sugar and carbohydrates that a person consumes are not used properly by his or her body. Sooner or later, the person's pancreas no longer produces insulin, creating high blood sugar, which can be very dangerous. According to the U.S. Department of Health and Human Services, more than twenty million people suffer from diabetes in this country.[1] Diabetes can lead to heart and kidney disease, stroke, blindness, hypertension, and death.

IS SUGAR AFFECTING YOUR HEALTH?

Take this short quiz to see if your sugar consumption may be affecting your level of health not only now but in the future as well:

Y/N Do you have a family history of diabetes?

Y/N Do you crave sweets at certain times of the day?

Y/N Do you crave sweets when you are under stress?

Y/N Do you consume ice cream, chocolate, pies, cakes, and candy more than twice a week?

Y/N Do you feel weak and shaky if your meal is delayed?

Y/N Do you feel tense, uptight, and nervous at certain times during the day?

Y/N Do you crave sodas or other sweetened soft drinks?

Y/N Do you choose low-fat foods while ignoring the higher sugar content typically found in them?

In addition to diabetes, excessive sugar consumption leads to high cholesterol and triglycerides (increasing the risk of atherosclerosis), excessive mood swings and food cravings (especially for women before menstruation), tooth decay, and gum disease.

Even small blood sugar fluctuations disturb a person's sense of well-being. Large fluctuations caused by consuming too much sugar cause feelings of depression, anxiety, mood swings, fatigue, and even aggressive behavior.

By combining low glycemic foods, such as fiber foods, together with exercise, amino acid supplementation, and nutritional supplements that help balance your blood sugar, you can optimize your brain's biochemistry.

The eating plan in chapter 6 has your blood sugar in mind. You will notice that stevia, a natural sweetener, has been substituted for sugar. Stevia is safe for diabetics and hypoglycemics. You will also notice that artificial sweeteners are nowhere to be found. This is because they have been implicated in very serious side effects. To satisfy your occasional sweet tooth without the health risks of artificial sweeteners, you can also substitute (if your health permits) the following: honey, rice syrup, sucarat (a natural sweetener made from sugar cane juice; use with caution if you have a blood sugar imbalance), or fructose (sugar derived from fruit).

A HIDDEN CAUSE OF FATIGUE

If you suffer from fatigue, you may have an iodine deficiency. A lack of iodine can impair your thyroid function, and a sluggish thyroid can leave you feeling tired and weak.

Luckily, there's an excellent test you can do at home to check your iodine levels. Simply take a Q-tip, dip it into a 2 percent tincture of iodine (available at any drugstore or supermarket), and paint a two-inch square on your thigh or belly. This will leave a yellowish stain on your skin that should disappear in about twenty-four hours if your iodine levels are normal.

If the stain disappears in *less* than twenty-four hours, that means your body is deficient in iodine and it has thirstily sucked it up. If that seems to be the case, keep applying the iodine every day at different sites on your body until the stain begins to last a full twenty-four hours.

Not only will you have diagnosed your iodine deficiency, you will also have treated that deficiency and improved your thyroid function! If you suspect poor thyroid function, you should ask your doctor to check your thyroid levels to determine whether or not you need to address the situation further.

FOOD ALLERGIES AND FATIGUE

Many people who complain of fatigue, depression, bloating, intestinal gas, nasal congestion, postnasal drip, and wheezing may suffer from a food sensitivity. Food allergies and sensitivities, especially the common allergies to dairy products and wheat, can cause digestive disturbances and poor absorption of nutrients, which result in more fatigue. Ninety percent of food allergies and sensitivities involve the following foods: milk, eggs, peanuts, tree nuts (such as cashews and walnuts), fish, shellfish, soy, and wheat.[2] To see if your problems with fatigue involve food allergies, you might decide to experiment with your diet.

Most often the culprit is dairy. Dairy products are one of the primary sources of food allergies in the standard American diet. Delayed reactions such as mood swings, dizziness, headaches, and joint pain can occur. When you add the fact that hormones and pesticides are used in livestock feed, cow's milk is not a healthy choice. Another important consideration is lactose, which is the predominant sugar in milk and which cannot be digested by many people.

The good news is that there are wonderful dairy substitutes that are full of calcium and are easy to assimilate. Try soy milk, rice milk, or almond milk. Try sorbet or other frozen desserts made from rice milk. Make smoothies with soy milk, rice milk, or almond milk. Try soy, almond, or rice cheese. Your body will quickly let you know that you have made a healthier choice. You may be able to watch all of your allergic symptoms disappear in about seven to fourteen days.

WHEAT ALLERGY DIET[3]

Foods made with wheat are staples of the American diet. The proteins found in wheat are collectively referred to as "gluten." Below are examples of wheat products and products that may contain wheat:

Wheat products:	
Whole wheat or enriched flour	Durum
High-gluten flour	Semolina
High-protein flour	Wheat malt
Bran	Wheat starch
Farina	Modified starch
Graham flour	Starch
Bulgur	

Foods made with wheat:	
Breads, cookies, cakes, and other baked goods made with wheat flour	Couscous
Bread crumbs	Cracker meal
Crackers	Pasta
Many cereals	Spelt
Acker meal	

Ingredients to look for:	
Gluten	Wheat germ
Gelatinized starch	Wheat gluten
Hydrolyzed vegetable protein	Vegetable gum
Vital gluten	Vegetable starch
Wheat bran	

Diet tip: Read all product labels carefully. Many processed foods, including ice cream and ketchup, may contain wheat flour. If you have a wheat allergy, you may try substituting flours and other products made from oats, rice, rye, barley, or corn.

Juicing

Have you ever tried juicing? You can obtain extra benefits from freshly juiced fruits and vegetables because juices are digested and assimilated within ten to fifteen minutes after you consume them, unlike raw fruits and vegetables, and they are used almost completely by your body to nourish and regenerate your cells, tissues, glands, and organs.

Specific juice recipes can target specific conditions. Since carrots (and yams) can help improve your resistance to allergies, try carrot juice by itself or in tasty combination with spinach, beets, and cucumbers. These juices have the added benefit of boosting your energy. They are fatigue-targeting juices.

Supplementation

To banish your fatigue for good, nutritional supplements may be required. The right supplements are part of every nutrient foundational protocol, and they should be tailored to your specific needs, which may change over time.

Always remember, the food you eat is *fuel*. It should energize you, not sideline you with fatigue and bloating. Enzyme supplementation can help you assimilate your food more efficiently. You may find that chronic allergies and chronic fatigue will disappear after you begin enzyme supplementation.

While it is possible to receive enzymes from raw foods that you eat, such as mangoes, papayas, bananas, avocados, and pineapples, I strongly suggest that you make sure you are "enzymatically insured" by supplementing your body with digestive enzymes from a plant source. Plant enzymes support digestion. Plant-based enzymes are considered to be the most effective because they have the ability to function under the entire range of gastric pHs that occur throughout your entire digestive system.

An ideal plant-based enzyme formula should contain the following:

- Protease (digests protein)
- Amylase (digests starches)
- Lipase (digests fats)
- Lactase (digests milk sugar)
- Cellulase (digests plant fiber)

- Invertase (digests refined sugar)
- Phytase (breaks down phytic acid)

The usual recommendation is to take two plant enzymes at the beginning of every meal. Be sure to stay well hydrated by drinking water every two hours whether you are thirsty or not. Pure water will help all of your body's systems to work more efficiently. In addition, water will lessen arthritic pain, help transport nutrients for assimilation, and help with proper elimination, removing toxins in the process.

TIRED AND TOXIC?

In other words, although you may find this hard to believe, sometimes your fatigue will yield to one of the simplest protocols of all—drinking more water. Lack of adequate water is often behind this common complaint. In our society, we consume gallons of coffee and liters of soft drinks and iced tea, and many people consider plain old water to be plain boring.

Water makes up 65 to 75 percent of your body. It is second only to oxygen for your survival. When you drink plenty of water, you flush out waste and toxins, regulate your body temperature, and improve the shock-absorbing ability of your joints, bones, and muscles. Water cleanses the body inside and out. It transports nutrients, proteins, vitamins, minerals, and sugars for assimilation. When you drink enough water, your body works at its peak.

Oddly enough, sometimes ingesting more water can solve a problem with water retention. Is part of your fatigue because of the sluggishness of edema and bloating? Drink more water. Is part of your fatigue because you are overweight and are you trying to lose some of that extra weight? Drink more water. Drinking water will curtail your hunger.

Add a few drops of lemon juice to increase the value of a glass of good, clean water. Sometimes the added taste is just what you need to help make it easier for you to change your habits and drink more water.

DETOXIFICATION

From time to time, you may need to take it a step farther. Many people who experience fatigue are suffering from the accumulated effects of toxins in their bodies. Their headaches, aches and pains, sinus problems, weight problems, foggy-headed feelings, intestinal gas, irregularity, indigestion, and mood swings may be warning signs that indicate a need for detoxification.

The world around us exposes us to pollution, and our food choices have filled us with chemicals from processed foods, not to mention sugar and caffeine. We have taken more medications than we realize, and often we have not eaten with any sort of balance due to our hectic lifestyles. We have neglected to eat enough fresh fruits and vegetables to provide us with the fiber that could move toxins out of our systems. Here we have the makings of autointoxication (self-poisoning). This occurs when the toxic buildup is so great that it recycles and enters the bloodstream, causing a myriad of uncomfortable symptoms that can baffle even the very best physicians.

Clearing the toxins from your body is a self-care procedure that can give us a fresh start every time we do it. Some people do it regularly twice a year, in the spring and in the fall, like "spring cleaning." The easiest, most user-friendly way to do this is to purchase an herbal formula that contains time-tested synergistic herbs that are system specific, meaning herbs that cleanse the liver, blood, colon, etc. When you take ancient herbal wisdom and marry it with the formulating technology of today, you have the benefit of having a very efficient way to correct toxic overload and regain your health.

When it comes to detoxification, there are other ways to go besides herbal formulations: colonics, fasting, saunas, enemas, and juicing, for instance. For ease, convenience, and effectiveness, herbal cleansing has been found to be the most effective, provided you use a superior product.

Whatever product you choose, remember that formulation is key. It must not be too harsh, and it must not consist of laxative herbs only. Find a formulation that contains the system-specific herbs as well as herbs that help sweep the colon for removal of toxins from your system. The process usually takes thirty to ninety days to gently eliminate years of accumulated waste matter. To further enhance the process, make sure that you clean up your diet and drink plenty of good-quality water.

After detoxification, many people feel as if they have been given their health back. Their skin clears up, their elimination is regular, their eyes sparkle, their energy soars, their vitality returns, their digestion improves, their aches and pains diminish or disappear, headaches become a thing of the past, and unhealthy cravings disappear.

Needless to say, after detoxification you must take a measure of responsibility and do your part to help prevent a recurring accumulation of toxins in your body.

INSOMNIA AND YOUR DIET

Sleep is a supreme tonic. It is important that you take steps to sleep deeply and restoratively. If you have trouble getting to sleep at night or trouble staying asleep all night long, you have insomnia. Lack of sleep robs your body of the essential downtime it needs to rebuild vital organs and recharge your nervous system. People who return from a restful vacation will say they feel rejuvenated. Friends and co-workers will usually comment on how rested and relaxed they appear. Good, sound, adequate amounts of sleep were probably part of their good vacation. Just think: if it is so evident on the outside, imagine what has taken place inside the person's body, mind, and spirit.

If you have insomnia, it is vital to determine and change the cause of it. It's not going to be enough to pop a pill at bedtime. If you are thinking of taking prescription sleep aids, you should know that sleeping pills impair calcium absorption, are habit forming, and may paralyze the part of your brain that controls dreaming. As a result, many times, sleeping pills can impair your clarity of thought and leave you feeling less than rested.

When you are working on reestablishing a healthy sleep pattern, take a hard look at your diet. Are you consuming caffeinated items such as coffee, tea, sodas, or chocolate? Are you consuming them in the evening? Caffeine is a stimulant, and it will keep you awake. What else are you consuming in the evening? It has been said that sleep doesn't interfere with digestion—but digestion does interfere with sleep!

If you are hungry in the late evening, choose a food that will promote relaxation. Here is a list of suggested foods (you will find further suggestions and more information in chapter 6 under "Sleep Inducers"):

- Plain yogurt
- A small bowl of oatmeal
- A small serving of lean turkey
- A banana
- A small serving of tuna
- A few whole-grain crackers

Unless you are concerned about the need to get up in the night to use the bathroom, you might want to try a cup of chamomile tea at bedtime. Chamomile is considered to be a nerve restorative that helps quiet anxiety and stress, probably because it is high in magnesium, calcium, potassium, and B vitamins.

Everybody thinks of turkey as a source of tryptophan when they think of a natural sleep inducer; you know how it gets blamed for those famous Thanksgiving afternoon naps. But tryptophan will work better when your stomach is *not* overstuffed as it might be on Thanksgiving, and it works better in combination with some complex carbohydrates. If you're about to go to bed, your body does not appreciate a protein overload. So if you are looking for the best midevening, sleep-promoting snack, take one slice of lean turkey and enjoy it on a slice of whole grain bread.

Natural Sleep Aids

- *Passionflower* helps to relax your mind and muscles. It is an antispasmodic sedative. You can take it in tincture form (30 drops) or capsule form (500 mg) thirty minutes before you turn in for the night.
- *Valerian* helps anxiety-related sleep disorders. Valerian has a strong odor that many people object to, so it is not usually desired as a tea. Some people may feel groggy or experience a "hangover effect" from valerian. If this happens to you, passionflower may be a better choice to help improve your sleep. Be careful not to combine valerian or passionflower with tranquilizers or antidepressant medications. Valerian also comes in tincture or capsule form. Take 30–60 drops or a 300–500 mg tablet thirty to sixty minutes before bedtime.

Several other natural supplements may also have beneficial effects:

- Hops: help to induce sleep and is a safe and reliable sedative
- Melatonin: a natural hormone that promotes sound sleep

- DHEA: a natural hormone that improves the quality of sleep
- L-theanine: an amino acid that, if taken thirty minutes before bed, promotes deep muscle relaxation
- Calcium: has a calming effect and, when combined with magnesium, feeds the nerves
- Magnesium: relaxes muscles and, with calcium, feeds the nerves
- Inositol: enhances REM (rapid eye movement) sleep, the stage of deep sleep at which dreaming occurs

You don't have to drag yourself through your life, low in mood as well as in energy. Stop compromising your health and banish fatigue for good.

chapter 5

DEPRESSION AND YOUR DIET

THE FIFTH CENTURY B.C. Greek physician Hippocrates, now known as the Father of Medicine, is often quoted as having said:

> From the brain, and from the brain only, arise our pleasures, joys, laughter, and jests, as well as our sorrows, pains, griefs, and tears.

Even two thousand five hundred years ago, well-informed people knew that a well-nourished brain would be more likely to be healthy and therefore able to keep your emotional state stable in spite of the stresses and difficulties of life. A person who is not depressed is more likely to eat a balanced diet, get adequate sleep, and undertake exercise, which all further contribute to his or her good health.

While imbalances can lead to depression, depression itself often leads to changes in appetite. Increased appetite can result in unwanted weight gain, which in turn can lead to increased risk of high blood pressure, diabetes, and heart disease. Decreased appetite can cause weight loss and reduced intake of essential nutrients. Both can lead to fatigue and a lack of resistance to disease.

Stormy emotions such as depression lead many people to overeat. When you are angry, irritable, resentful, unforgiving, and uptight, your levels of the stress hormone called *cortisol* become elevated. Cortisol stimulates your appetite because one of its main roles in the stress response is to refuel you with carbohydrates and fats after you have completed the fight-or-flight response. Here's the catch, though.

If you never complete the fight-or-flight response and you leave your emotional stress-response motor running, the result will be an insatiable appetite for sweets, the quick fix for stress relief. This quick fix, unfortunately, leads to a quick expansion of your waistline.

Changes in food intake might mean reduced levels of some nutrients that have been specifically linked to depression, thus intensifying the problem. In particular, deficiencies in the B vitamins—folic acid, thiamin, riboflavin, niacin, and B_6—can lead to a clinical depression. Iron-deficiency anemia can also lead to depression.

As we know, many health problems include a depression component. Whether the depression is rooted in a physical injury or illness or biochemical imbalance or whether it seems to be a person's primary health problem, it looms large on our screens.

SIGNS OF DEPRESSION

The many and varied symptoms of depression may include:

- A "slowdown" of physical movements
- Actual suicide attempts
- Changes in eating habits
- Changes in sleeping patterns
- Continually mulling over the past, reviewing your mistakes
- Difficulty making decisions
- Fatigue
- Feelings of emptiness
- Feelings of guilt
- Feelings of helplessness
- Feelings of hopelessness
- Feelings of pessimism
- Feelings of worthlessness
- Inability to concentrate
- Loss of interest in sex
- Loss of interest in usually pleasurable activities
- Loss of self-esteem
- Memory difficulties

SIGNS OF DEPRESSION

- Profound, persistent irritability
- Profound, persistent sadness
- Restlessness
- Thoughts of suicide or death
- Unexplained crying
- Unexplained headaches, stomach upsets, or other physical problems that are not helped with standard treatment
- Unexplained weight gain or loss

Depression can come from prolonged stress (sometimes caused by negative emotional behavior learned in childhood), which causes a deficiency of amino acids that results in a biochemical imbalance. When certain nutrients are not supplied to our brains, a set of negative emotions can cascade, and our ability to cope is compromised.

The answer is not just to take supplements, although as you will see in this chapter, it may be one of the best ways to supply the missing nutrients to your brain. If you follow my eating plan (See part 2 of this book, "How to Feel Your Best"), you will begin to resupply your depleted brain and body with the nutrients they need.

When you are consuming a balanced diet, you will become more able to control your cravings because your cortisol levels will not be elevated. You will be able to practice "nutritious noshing," meaning snacking on nutrient-dense foods that build your health without piling on the pounds.

Sometimes the smartest thing you can do for yourself is to take a break, relax, and prepare a high-protein shake for yourself. Your protein demands go up during stressful periods. Remember, amino acids are the building blocks of protein. Amino acids are crucial for brain health. If you are experiencing signs of depression, you should *avoid* alcohol, caffeine, and sugar, all of which cause changes in energy and mood.

BRING ON THE PROTEIN

After water, the second highest proportion of your body is composed of protein. It's in your muscles, your bones, your skin, your hair, and almost every other organ or tissue in your body—about 75 percent of your weight, minus the water weight, in fact. Whether you are aware of the fact or not, your body consists of at least ten thousand distinctly different proteins, without which you would not be alive and relatively healthy.[1]

Protein is all important. It comprises the enzymes in your body, without which all of those unseen chemical reactions could not take place. It's part of the hemoglobin that carries oxygen in your bloodstream.

Those ten thousand different proteins are built from about twenty different amino acids. Your body "knows" genetically how to combine these amino acids into proteins. Some are very complex, and some are simpler. To obtain the amino acids, you must eat or drink them in your food or beverages because your body cannot manufacture them, nor can they be stored in your body for future use.

As an adult, you need at least 9 grams of protein daily for every 20 pounds of body weight.[2] That protein can come from a number of dietary sources, and people disagree about which sources are best.

All protein sources are not equally valuable or accessible for your body's needs. Animal sources of protein (meat, fish, poultry, eggs, milk, and other dairy products) are what is known as "complete," because those sources contain all the amino acids needed to build proteins. Other protein sources lack one or more of the amino acids needed by your body in order to make new protein. Your body cannot make these missing amino acids itself, even by modifying another amino acid. So these protein sources are called "incomplete" because they do not furnish the complete package of amino acids. Fruits, vegetables, grains, and nuts furnish incomplete proteins. Vegetarians know about this, and they combine nonmeat and/or nondairy protein sources in order to furnish their bodies with the right assortment of amino acids.

A simple American diet furnishes more than enough protein. All you need is a bowl of breakfast cereal plus milk, a peanut butter and jelly sandwich for lunch, and a piece of fish with some beans for supper, and you have consumed about 70 grams of protein, which is more than enough for the average adult.[3]

In the United States, unlike in other parts of the world, we don't have any difficulty obtaining protein sources, although we sometimes have the opposite problem—too much of a good thing, which compromises our health in a number of ways. In the parts of the world where protein is scarce, it's the children who suffer the most. Their growing bodies need protein in order to become strong and stay healthy.

Without adequate protein, the human body loses muscle mass and suffers increasingly weakened cardiovascular and respiratory systems, decreased immunity, mental problems, and, ultimately, death.

The importance of protein for your mental health, not to mention your physical health, cannot be overemphasized.

DIETARY SOURCES OF PROTEIN[4]

Food	Serving	Weight in Grams	Protein Grams	% Daily Value
Hamburger, extra lean	6 oz.	170	48.6	97
Chicken, roasted	6 oz.	170	42.5	85
Fish	6 oz.	170	41.2	82
Tuna, water packed	6 oz.	170	40.1	80
Beefsteak, broiled	6 oz.	170	38.6	77
Cottage cheese	1 cup	225	28.1	56
Cheese pizza	2 slices	128	15.4	31
Yogurt, low fat	8 oz.	227	11.9	24
Tofu	½ cup	126	10.1	20
Lentils, cooked	½ cup	99	9	18
Skim milk	1 cup	245	8.4	17
Split peas, cooked	½ cup	98	8.1	16
Whole milk	1 cup	244	8	16
Lentil soup	1 cup	242	7.8	16
Kidney beans, cooked	½ cup	87	7.6	15
Cheddar cheese	1 oz.	28	7.1	14
Macaroni, cooked	1 cup	140	6.8	14
Soy milk	1 cup	245	6.7	13
Egg	1 large	50	6.3	13
Whole-wheat bread	2 slices	56	5.4	11

DIETARY SOURCES OF PROTEIN[4]

Food	Serving	Weight in Grams	Protein Grams	% Daily Value
White bread	2 slices	60	4.9	10
Rice, cooked	1 cup	158	4.3	9
Broccoli, cooked	5-inch piece	140	4.2	8
Baked potato	2x5 inches	156	3	6
Corn, cooked	1 ear	77	2.6	5

Choose a variety of low-fat sources of protein daily and eat modest servings. A normal serving of lean meat, poultry, or fish would be 2 or 3 ounces in weight (about the size of a pack of playing cards). An average portion size for cooked dry legumes or beans would be half a cup. One egg and 2 tablespoons of peanut butter count as 1 ounce of lean meat.

AMINO ACIDS: THE NATURAL TRANQUILIZERS

Once you have discovered that amino acids play a vital role in your brain's health, you will be ready to understand the important link between your brain and your emotions. Some amino acids act as major inhibitory neurotransmitters. The following amino acids help to restore and replenish your brain when you are feeling depressed or uptight:

- *Glutamine*—This amino acid is a prime brain nutrient and energy source. Supplementing your brain with glutamine can rapidly improve memory, recall, concentration, and alertness. It also helps to reduce sugar and alcohol cravings, and it controls hypoglycemic reactions.
- *Lysine*—This an essential amino acid is effective in the natural treatment of hypothyroidism, Alzheimer's disease, and Parkinson's disease.
- *Tyrosine*—This is a wonderful semiessential amino acid formed from phenylalanine. Tyrosine helps to build

the body's natural supply of adrenaline and thyroid hormones. It is also an antioxidant and a source of quick energy, especially for the brain. Because it converts in the body to the amino acid L-dopa, it is considered to be a safe, natural support for Parkinson's disease, depression, and hypertension. Avoid tyrosine if you have cancerous melanoma or manic depression.

- *Glycine*—This amino acid helps to release growth hormones when taken in large doses. It converts to creatine in the body to retard nerve and muscle degeneration. It is wonderful for controlling and regulating hypoglycemic symptoms, especially when taken in the morning upon rising.

- *Taurine*—A potent antiseizure amino acid, taurine is a neurotransmitter that helps to control the nervous system and hyperactivity. It also works to normalize irregular heartbeats, helps prevent circulatory and heart disorders, and helps to lower cholesterol. Since natural sources of taurine are hard to find, supplementation is the best way to receive adequate amounts for therapeutic benefit.

GUIDELINES FOR TAKING AMINO ACIDS

Take amino acids before meals with the exception of brain-stimulant amino acids.

Take amino acids with their nutrient cofactors for the best uptake.

Make sure to take amino acids with plenty of water for optimum absorption.

Note that active forms of amino acids are the only ones available for sale. Even if you do not see "L-" (which stands for levo) or "D-" (which stands for dextro) before the amino acid, the product is still in its active form. For example, L-carnitine and carnitine are the same.

The Big B Connection

Since this book is devoted to the connection between nutrition and your mood, I would be remiss if I did not discuss the importance of the B vitamins.

B vitamins dramatically affect proper functioning of your nervous system. I believe that B vitamins are the most influential factor in maintaining a healthy nervous system. When my clients are under stress of any kind, whether it is physical, emotional, or mental, I immediately recommend a good, total B complex. As you read on, you'll see why I recommend the B vitamins to help fend off overload and depression in times of stress.

B_1, commonly known as thiamine, is known as the "morale vitamin" because of its beneficial effect on your attitude. It is also crucial to the health of your nervous system. If your diet is high in carbohydrates, then B_1 is absolutely essential. B_1 improves food assimilation, thereby stabilizing your appetite. If you happen to be deficient in vitamin B_1, you may notice one or more of these symptoms: fatigue, loss of ankle and knee reflexes, mental instability, forgetfulness, fears, cardiac malfunctions such as rapid rhythm and palpitations, and inflammation of the optic nerve.

B_2, which is known as riboflavin, is a water-soluble vitamin that is easily absorbed through the small intestines. It plays an important part in any chemical reactions in the body, and it has been shown to be an inhibitor of tumor growth. B_2 deficiency symptoms include shiny tongue, eye burning and itching, feeling of sand or grit in eyes, oily skin, difficulty in urination, and scaly skin around mouth, nose, and ears.

Niacin, or B_3, assists in the functioning of your digestive system, and it helps to maintain the health of your skin and nerves. It is important for the conversion of food to energy.

B_6 should not be taken by itself; it must be taken with amino acids. You may take a B-complex formula that contains B_6 and the full spectrum of B vitamins. B_6 may have the greatest effect on the immune system of all the B vitamins, because a deficiency can result in a vast array of immune-response problems and has been linked to tumor growth. A lack of B_6 makes the size of the thymus—the gland that produces T cells—decrease in size.

B$_{12}$ is also known as cobalamin, and on the molecular level, it is the most complex of all the B group. It is required by your body for the formation of red blood cells, which are needed to prevent mood-sapping fatigue and low energy. Vitamin B$_{12}$ is crucial too for your body because it helps your system process fats.

Neither humans nor animals can manufacture B$_{12}$ in their bodies, which must be combined with calcium for proper absorption. Many people have a hard time absorbing B$_{12}$ from the foods they eat, and vegetarian foods are lacking in this important vitamin, so I recommend that everyone take a daily doses of B-complex in order to obtain the B$_{12}$ they need. When B$_{12}$ is deficient, anemia can occur along with sore tongue, weight loss, mental deterioration, menstrual disturbances, and a "needles-and-pins" sensation.

Pantothenic acid, also called biotin or B$_5$, is a blessing when a person is under stress. It has an enhancing and beneficial effect upon the adrenal glands, whose proper functioning is crucial when a person is under stressful conditions.

GETTING B VITAMINS FROM YOUR FOOD[5]

Food sources for vitamin B$_1$ (thiamine):	Thiamine is found in fortified breads, cereals, pasta, whole grains (especially wheat germ), lean meats (especially pork), fish, dried beans, peas, and soybeans. Dairy products, fruits, and vegetables are not very high in thiamine, but when consumed in large amounts, they become a significant source.
Food sources for vitamin B$_2$ (riboflavin):	Lean meats, eggs, legumes, nuts, green leafy vegetables, dairy products, and milk provide riboflavin in the diet. Breads and cereals are often fortified with riboflavin. Because riboflavin is destroyed by exposure to light, foods with riboflavin should not be stored in glass containers that are exposed to light.

GETTING B VITAMINS FROM YOUR FOOD[5]

Food sources for vitamin B_3 (niacin):	Niacin is found in dairy products, poultry, fish, lean meats, nuts, and eggs. Legumes and enriched breads and cereals also supply some niacin.
Food sources for vitamin B_6:	Vitamin B_6 is found in beans, nuts, legumes, eggs, meats, fish, whole grains, and fortified breads and cereals.
Food sources for vitamin B_5 (pantothenic acid, biotin):	Pantothenic acid and biotin are found in foods that are good sources of B vitamins, including the following: eggs, fish, milk and milk products, whole-grain cereals, legumes, yeast, broccoli and other vegetables in the cabbage family, white and sweet potatoes, and lean beef.
Food sources for vitamin B_{12}:	Vitamin B_{12} is found in eggs, meat, poultry, shellfish, and milk and milk products.

OTHER SUPPLEMENTS

As you develop your own personal mood-boosting plan, you will want to consider the following supplements. (These are available at your local health food store, except where I've directed you to the product list in Appendix B.)

GABA

You will find GABA (gamma-aminobutyric acid) mentioned throughout this book. This is because the amino acid GABA affects your mood, your memory, and your behavior. GABA has a natural calming effect, and it helps to cool the brain. Remember that amino acid deficiencies occur when we experience long periods of pain, stress, trauma, depression, or anxiety. Because coping with taxing circumstances depletes your supply of GABA, I recommend that you take it as a supplement. Once depletion occurs, your brain becomes overwhelmed by anxiety signals, leaving you tense and out of control.

Your brain needs more than 100 mg of GABA to restore the proper level. I recommend capsules over tablets for easier assimilation. (This is true for all of my supplement recommendations.)

Liquid serotonin

If you are not currently taking a prescription SSRI medication (commonly known as selective serotonin reuptake inhibitors), you may take liquid serotonin. Serotonin is a key neurotransmitter in brain function that enhances focus, elevates mood, and reduces anger and aggression. It can also help reduce cravings for carbohydrates and alcohol.

Magnesium gelcaps

Low magnesium levels are found in persons with hyperirritability, depression, and anxiety. I recommend that you take 400 mg at bedtime. Magnesium also helps your muscles to relax.

Brain Link and Anxiety Control 24

Brain Link is the name of a total amino-acid complex that blankets your system with all of the amino acids that create neurotransmitter links for enhanced brain function. It comes in powder form and can be mixed with juice for daily use. Brain Link contains the major inhibitory neurotransmitters, GABA, glutamine, and glycine and is safe for children and adults. (See Appendix B for more information.)

Anxiety Control 24 is a patented amino acid support formula that contains amino acids, herbs, vitamins, and minerals, along with essential cofactors to help relax the anxious mind or stressed body. It contains magnesium, vitamin B_6, GABA, glycine, glutamine, and the herbs passionflower and *primula officanalis*. (See Appendix B for more information.)

Don't wait until you're too depressed to make changes in your nutritional habits. When you first realize that you are struggling with depression, resist the temptation to resort to foods and other substances that will only intensify your chemical imbalance. Eat smart from the start, and you may not need to seek further help. If you do need supplemental support, your good nutritional habits will make your return to happiness a smoother one.

PART 2

HOW TO FEEL YOUR BEST

EACH AND EVERY one of us wants to feel our best at all times. It makes such a huge difference in life. Even a child knows that if he or she is in a bad mood, "nothing goes right." By contrast, when you're in a *good* mood, the sky can be falling and yet you're able to handle the fallout with composure.

Quite simply, the most basic, fundamental, foundational component of feeling your very best is consuming personally balanced nutrition every single day. Each person is a little different, although there are certain common denominators, so you need to explore both the principles and the possibilities as you come up with a manageable, affordable, and sustainable nutrition plan that works for *you*.

chapter 6

THE FEEL-GOOD DIET PROGRAM

WHEN YOU ARE struggling with a low mood, you feel drained in every way—emotionally, mentally, and physically. It's bad enough to feel this way. What's worse is that when you feel bad, you fail to care for yourself. You can't do it. Taking care of yourself requires *energy*, one of the qualities you are having a hard time maintaining. Not caring for yourself means you stay pretty much where you are, with a low mood, sluggish mind, and a body with an increasing number of physical complaints.

MEAL PLAN

It is so important to make a conscious effort to eat properly, because your body needs high-quality fuel in order to repair, rebuild, and regenerate itself. In the United States, many of the foods we prefer, instead of being high-quality sources of nutrition, actually sabotage our physical health, not to mention our emotional health.

This eating plan is high in nutrition, yet it eliminates all the foods that can lower both your mood and your physical and mental health.

THE EATING PLAN

On rising:	One 8-ounce glass of water with juice from ½ of a fresh lemon (you may add stevia extract to sweeten). Add 1 teaspoon of apple cider vinegar if you have flatulence.
Breakfast:	(Choose one of the following.) One or two poached or hard-boiled eggs on a slice of millet bread Oatmeal or oat bran with 1 tablespoon Braggs Aminos Buckwheat pancakes with a little butter or almond butter Millet toast with almond butter
Midmorning snack:	(Choose one of the following.) A glass of a green drink (liquid chlorophyll or Kyo-Green) A cup of dandelion tea A small bottle of water
Lunch:	(Choose one of the following.) A fresh green salad with lemon and olive oil dressing An open-faced millet sandwich with mayonnaise, veggies, seafood, turkey, or chicken Vegetable soup with a piece of millet bread Chicken, tuna, or vegetable pasta salad
Midafternoon snack:	(Choose one of the following.) Rice crackers or baked corn chips with some rice cheese or soy cheese A bottle of water with a hard-boiled or deviled egg Raw veggies And: A cup of green tea with stevia to sweeten

Dinner:	(Choose one of the following.)
	Baked, broiled, or poached fish or chicken or turkey with steamed brown rice
	Baked potato with Bragg Aminos
	Rice with soy cheese
	Oriental stir-fry with brown rice and Braggs Aminos
	A small omelet with a veggie filling (soy or rice cheese can be added)
	Vegetarian casserole
	A hot or cold vegetable pasta salad
Before bed:	A cup of herbal tea such as dandelion or chamomile with stevia* to sweeten

RECOMMENDED SUPPLEMENTS

Here is a list of the supplements I've mentioned above. These supplements are available at your local health food store:

1. *Kyo-Green*: A complete green superfood that contains protein and all the B vitamins. It heals the intestinal tract, strengthens the liver, and boosts immune health. It is a good detoxifier and blood cleanser rich in chlorophyll.

2. *Stevia extract*: Also known as "sweet herb" (*stevia rebaudiana*), this is a South American sweetening leaf. Stevia is twenty-five times sweeter than sugar, and yet it balances the blood sugar and has antifungal properties. It also has zero calories. Unlike sugar, it does not promote tooth decay. You can make delicious lemonade with fresh lemons, water, and stevia extract to taste. Drink it throughout the day to keep your blood sugar stable.

3. *Braggs Amino Acids*: This product is a natural health alternative to soy sauce. Made from soybeans and purified water only (no additives, preservatives, alcohol, or chemicals), it can be dashed or sprayed on salads, vegetables, rice and beans, tofu, casseroles, soups,

potatoes, meats, fish, poultry, jerky, tempeh, gravies, sauces, and popcorn.

MIND MEDICINES

GABA

GABA (gamma-aminobutyric acid) is a naturally occurring amino acid. Natural substances cannot be patented and therefore do not create profits large enough to drive a large-scale marketing operation. Nevertheless, GABA supplementation is often the first choice for people who want to restore the natural balance within their bodies and minds.

GABA actually fills the GABA receptor sites in the brain while drugs merely attach to the receptors. Proponents believe that by restoring the brain chemistry with GABA and other amino acids, the brain becomes balanced. This is much more desirable than merely suppressing unpleasant symptoms with the anxiety drug *du jour*. Life is meant to be fully lived, with all of your senses sharp, clear, and intact. Prozac, Zoloft, Paxil, and Effexor suppress all your feelings, not only the unpleasant ones. They are "equal-opportunity mood suppressors" and they do not discriminate between pain, fear, happiness, or depression. They block excitatory messages as well as use your available serotonin, which affects your mood and your perception of pain. When your emotions are suppressed by medication, it's difficult to function at work or home.

In a sense, medication causes you to live life from within a dull cloud. If you choose to supplement with natural amino acids such as GABA, your root problem can be corrected. Your mind and senses will not be dulled, and you will not have to worry about becoming addicted.

When your brain is provided with adequate amounts of amino acids, which are the building blocks for neurotransmitters, your behavior is normal. If you are deficient, you may have a constant anxiety problem.

When the GABA supply is deficient, your brain suffers and your body is flooded with uncomfortable, life-disrupting symptoms. You can overhaul your entire nutritional regimen and yet continue to have mood swings and disconcerting mental and physical symptoms—all because of a GABA deficiency. Over and over in my practice, I have recommended GABA to my clients with excellent results. GABA proved to be invaluable in their quest for emotional balance and freedom from anxiety and other stress-related ailments.

Traumatic memories can be stored throughout your body. Your brain is not the only organ that suffers. Your stomach, skin, muscles, heart, skeletal system, and any other organ of your body can "remember" a stressful experience as well. Since GABA receptors occur throughout your entire body, it is believed that taking GABA in the proper amounts can help to reduce the stress and tension throughout your body.

When your GABA supply has been depleted, your entire body will tell you about it:

- *Eyes*—your pupils dilate, you have blurred vision.
- *Mouth*—you have a dry mouth, perhaps a choking sensation.
- *Heart*—your heart races, or you have palpitations, pounding.
- *Lungs*—you have difficulty breathing because your bronchioles constrict.
- *Stomach*—your stomach contracts and you suffer from nausea and indigestion.
- *Adrenal glands*—your adrenals release adrenaline; you end up with no energy and are weak.
- *Colon*—you have gas, diarrhea, and constipation.
- *Bladder*—you have frequent urination.

TRAUMA DEPLETES GABA

Emotions that deplete GABA include:

Anger
Anxiety
Fear
Grief
Pain
Panic

TRAUMA DEPLETES GABA

Unresolved emotions lead to chronic pain, illness, and other physical symptoms. In addition, the following anxiety-related symptoms appear:

Back pain
Crying
Difficulty breathing
Headaches
Insomnia
Neck pain
Panic attacks
Rapid heartbeat

GABA is the main inhibitory neurotransmitter that restores your brain, functioning to regulate anxiety, moods, muscle spasms, depression, and chronic stress. For its proper metabolism, other nutrients work along with GABA.

Magnesium

One of those helpful nutrients is magnesium. Magnesium is a mineral that enhances GABA's action and effect on your body. Interestingly, most people with long-standing anxiety and stress problems are deficient in magnesium. You will note that the symptoms of magnesium deficiency are the same as those that occur with anxiety, stress, and emotional depletion.

SYMPTOMS OF MAGNESIUM DEFICIENCY

Anxiety	Irregular heartbeat
Asthma	Irritable bowel syndrome
Chronic pain	Low blood sugar
Constipation	Mitral valve prolapse
Depression	

SYMPTOMS OF MAGNESIUM DEFICIENCY

Dizziness	Muscle spasms
Fatigue	Noise sensitivity
Fibromyalgia	Panic attacks
Headaches	Spastic symptoms

According to many different experts, while GABA replenishment can replace some of the most overprescribed medications of our day, such as Prozac, Xanax, Valium, and other mood-altering drugs, magnesium enhances the effect of the replenishment even more.

When you are chronically stressed, you can become magnesium deficient, even if you eat foods that are rich in magnesium daily. This is because in addition to becoming irritable, easily fatigued, and muddled in your thinking, chronic stress makes your blood pressure increase. Under these conditions, magnesium is released from your blood cells and goes into your blood plasma. From there it is excreted in your urine.

To turn this around, you need to take at least 400 mg of magnesium at bedtime.

MAGNESIUM-RICH FOODS

You should also add the following magnesium-rich foods to your diet:

Almonds	Kidney beans
Bananas	Millet
Blackberries	Navy beans
Black-eyed peas	Shrimp
Broccoli	Soybeans
Dates	Watermelon
Green beans	Tuna
Kasha (buckwheat)	

Progesterone

Progesterone is important to your central nervous system. It is concentrated in brain cells in levels twenty times higher than that of blood serum levels. This indicates that it must serve some vital purpose.

Progesterone has a calming or mildly sedating effect on your brain. You will remember that GABA is a neurotransmitter inhibitor that has a calming effect as well. Do you see why both substances can help balance your mood swings and anxiety? This information is particularly helpful for women who are in the premenopause or menopause stage of life. Progesterone can balance out the roller-coaster ride of hot flashes, irritability, mood swings, headaches, fatigue, foggy thinking, and more. In addition, it can help alleviate anxiety and the nervous symptoms associated with this season of life. See the Product Sources appendix at the back of this book for my own Dr. Janet's Balanced by Nature Progesterone Cream.

Other amino acids

In chapter 1, "The Mind-Body Connection," I listed several amino acids, in addition to GABA and magnesium, that are "natural tranquilizers." They are, for your review, as follows:

- Glutamine
- Lysine
- Tyrosine
- Glycine
- Taurine

By now, you can see that I am a strong believer in the value of depending upon your own God-created mood-balancing system, which is built upon a strong foundation of natural mood-stabilizing amino acids.

BRAIN BALANCERS

If you want to keep your mental edge and steer clear of roller-coaster moods, your brain needs continual attention. Make sure that you are feeding your brain all of the nutrients it needs to function at optimal levels. By taking care of your brain now, you will safeguard yourself from the mental deterioration that can come from the aging process.

Exercise is another lesson in the mind-body connection. A fit body contributes to a fit mind. Any type of exercise performed at least three times a week will help keep you fit. Exercise keeps your blood well supplied with oxygen by increasing your lung capacity and conditioning your heart. This will supercharge your brain. Exercise also causes your brain to produce more nerve growth factor, or NGF. Nerve growth factor helps brain cells to create branches that connect to fellow brain cells, so that information can be transferred speedily and accurately.

Over time, your brain does not produce as many neurotransmitters as it once did. So supplementation becomes very important as you age, especially when you experience stress.

Omega-3 fatty acids and your moods

A Harvard study showed that omega-3 fatty acids can help reduce bad moods. Additional studies point out that consuming omega-3 fats can improve scores on psychological tests.[1] In addition, omega-3 fatty acids and other essential fatty acids improve the health of your cardiovascular system, your nervous system, your skin health, your fat metabolism, and your joint flexibility. (They're not called "essential" fatty acids for nothing!)

The typical American diet does not supply the proper essential fatty acids on its own, so you must supplement your diet with them. Look for supplements that supply omega-3 and omega-6 oils derived from fish oil, flax oil, or borage oil. Please note that even though you will find most of these fatty acids in dark containers to keep out the light, they may go rancid quickly. This is especially true for flaxseed oil. If you cannot use a bottle of fish oil in a month, then purchase a smaller bottle (and keep it in the refrigerator) or stick with capsules.

Other brain/mood helpers

In chapter 5, I discussed the role that the B vitamins play in helping you to maintain peak brain health. Other supplements provide distinct benefits.

Ginkgo

Ginkgo enhances neurotransmitter production and helps your brain use glucose for energy production. Another bonus is that ginkgo improves the flow of blood through your brain's tiny capillaries, which in turn increases your brain's supply of oxygen and glucose. Ginkgo can help offset ordinary memory loss when it is taken over a three-month period. Tinnitus (ringing in the ears) has also been helped or alleviated by using ginkgo. Ginkgo is not recommended, however, if you are taking blood thinners of any kind, because it may enhance their effect.

Phosphatidyl serine (PS)

PS helps to transmit nerve impulses from one cell to another. It has been found to be useful in various types of memory loss.

Acetyl-L-carnitine (ALC)

ALC helps to ease depression and helps cells fight free radicals and burn fat for energy.

Huperzine A

Huperzine A is derived from Chinese moss, and it helps your brain hang on to acetylcholine, which is a neurotransmitter vital to memory. A Chinese study found that huperzine A improved the mental functioning of Alzheimer's patients.

BRAIN/MOOD BALANCE AT A GLANCE

To strengthen your body in times of stress:	Astragalus Jiaogulan Siberian ginseng Suma
To help calm your mind:	Kava Passionflower
To feed your adrenal glands:	B-complex vitamins Liquid chlorophyll (such as Kyo-Green) Pantothenic acid Royal jelly

HORMONE HELPERS

As I indicated earlier, both the hormone progesterone (in its natural form) and GABA (gamma-aminobutyric acid) have a calming effect on your brain. Progesterone is essential for the health of your central nervous system, and it is concentrated in your brain cells in levels that are twenty times higher than your blood serum levels.[2] This strongly suggests that progesterone in brain cells must serve a very important purpose.

The calming or mildly sedating effect of progesterone may be caused directly by the hormone, or it may be caused by substances created from progesterone that are active at GABA receptor sites. GABA is a neurotransmitter inhibitor that has a calming effect also.

In my own case, supplementing my body's depleted progesterone resulted not only in rebalancing my severe hormonal imbalance, but it also helped to calm my anxious mind and to promote a sense of well-being. When I added GABA to my health-building protocol, the difference was truly amazing. This combination is particularly helpful for women who are going through perimenopause or menopause.

PMS program

In chapter 2, "Hormones and Your Diet," I gave the following guidelines for optimizing a woman's premenopausal health.

Your diet should be low in fat, and it should include regular seafood consumption. Be sure to eat plenty of cruciferous vegetables (broccoli, cauliflower) and dark, leafy greens to reduce estrogen buildup. Prepare brown rice often to obtain B vitamins. As much as possible, purchase organic meats, milk and milk products, and canned foods. Eliminate dairy products completely during your premenstrual days. Choose whole-grain food products, and keep your diet low in sugar and salt. Avoid caffeine and animal products as much as possible. Add fiber to your diet and drink plenty of water to keep your bowel function regular. Split your daily meals into many small meals eaten throughout the day.

To help control premenstrual cravings for sweets (mainly chocolate and refined sugar), increased appetite, headaches, and fatigue, consider supplementing your diet with a daily balanced B-complex vitamin, chromium picolinate, calcium, and magnesium.

To ease your water retentiveness (which is why you have breast tenderness, bloating, and headaches), eliminate caffeine and chocolate. You can also use evening primrose oil and ginkgo biloba. To relieve lower back pain, take quercetin or bromelain, or use ginger packs.

These recommendations may take two or three full monthly cycles to take full effect. You will need to be consistent in applying the changes to your diet in order to maintain your improvement.

Menopausal program

The unpleasant symptoms of perimenopause and menopause include mood swings, fatigue, breast tenderness, foggy thinking, irritability, headaches, insomnia, decreased sex drive, anxiety, depression, allergy symptoms (including asthma), fat gain (especially around the middle), hair loss, memory loss, water retention, bone loss, slow metabolism, endometrial and breast cancers, and many more. In other words, hormonal imbalance has far-reaching effects on many tissues in the body, including the heart, brain, blood vessels, bones, uterus, and breasts.

If you are a perimenopausal woman, besides adding a progesterone cream to your daily regimen you might want to consider the following supplements (described in more detail in chapter 2, "Hormones and Your Diet"): quercetin (a potent antioxidant), chaste tree berry (for progesterone production), bromelain, flaxseed oil (to help increase your intake of essential fatty acids), and vitamin C.

If you are already menopausal (meaning you have ceased having monthly periods), you may have noticed your tendency to gain weight. Conquer your appetite along with your nutrition, and you will be miles ahead. Naturally, your hormonal depletion has become noticeable as well, and you can incorporate some nutritional substitutes to help balance your body's ups and downs. In other words, you can get some hormonal help from plant sources that you include in your regular diet. Soybeans, black cohosh, Mexican wild yam, and licorice can be of benefit to a perimeno-pausal/menopausal woman. For many women, stressful lifestyles have made it necessary to move up to bioidentical hormones that are derived from these plants and then synthesized in a lab to be molecularly similar to the hormones our bodies make—estrogen, progesterone, DHEA, and so forth. This is unlike synthetic hormones, which are patented under names such as Prempro, Provera, and Premarin. Bioidentical hormones are much safer for your body because they are easier for your body to metabolize without many of the side effects that synthetic hormones create.

Neither bioidentical hormones nor synthetic hormones can do the whole job alone. You must address your diet and lifestyle, eating sensibly, drinking plenty of water, taking a calcium supplement and a good daily multivitamin, and getting plenty of rest.

You should follow these dietary guidelines (listed for you also in chapter 2) to help ease the symptoms of menopause:

- Add soy foods to your diet.
- Limit sugar, caffeine, pies, cakes, and pastries.
- Limit red meat.
- Eat fresh vegetables, fruits, and nuts.
- Instead of three large meals a day, eat several smaller meals throughout the day.
- Limit dairy products.

There are also many natural herbal remedies that can alleviate your menopause symptoms and help you find balance in this season of life. I suggest that you try them one by one and determine for yourself the ones that really give you comfort:

- Black cohosh
- Dong quai (high in phytoestrogens)
- Bioflavonoids (also high in phytoestrogens)
- Black currant seed oil
- Licorice (for your adrenal health)
- Plant enzymes (taken with meals)
- Red raspberry
- Vitamin B-complex
- Vitamin C
- Vitamin E (normalizes hormones)
- 5-HTP (5-hydroxytryptophan, for insomnia and anxiety at night)

STRESS BUSTERS

A certain level of stress is a normal and expected part of life, but when stress is severe, long lasting, or happens too frequently, our health will be jeopardized. Here are some powerful stress busters to help you create a foundation of good health:

1. *Eat well.* Apply what you have learned in this book and from your own experience to gain the benefits of eating well. What is best for you? Besides choosing foods that are health producing, make meals a pleasant social time. Make menu planning, table setting, cooking, eating, and even dish washing enjoyable times with family and friends. Eating the right foods in the right quantities will keep you well enough to face distressing challenges.

2. *Sleep deeply* every night. Sound sleep is essential for maintaining your emotional health and a healthy immune system. Most people don't get enough sleep. Find out how much you need by sleeping without being awakened by an alarm clock for a period of time. When you awake naturally, don't you feel relaxed? If you have trouble

falling asleep, establish a regular evening routine that does not include vigorous exercise or caffeine, adjusting your bedtime no more than an hour on weekends.

3. *Confide in a friend.* In times of stress, you need to be able to talk about your problems with someone who is concerned about you. It's important for you to be able to express yourself, to know that someone wants to hear about you. Laugh together too, because laughter releases tension. Laugh about everyday things or watch a classic comedy together.

4. *Express yourself* in creative ways. Do you have a hobby? Indulge in it—painting, gardening, dancing, writing in a journal, refinishing furniture, playing a musical instrument, or singing with a group or when you're alone.

5. *Simplify* your life. Take inventory of how you spend your time, money, and energy and decide whether you really want to continue doing all of those things. If you stop doing something, will you or your family suffer—or benefit? If you are overextended, learn to use the magic word *no.* Find joy in the simple things; make time to stop and smell the roses.

6. *Exercise* your body. Regular exercise is a natural releaser of stress. Exercise enhances your mood. The increased circulation of your blood increases your general immune protection and at the same time helps buffer the immunosuppression of distress. Exercise makes your body more fit for handling physical challenges. It doesn't have to be in a gym or structured in any way, unless that's what you prefer. You can work exercise into your daily life by taking the stairs instead of the elevator, parking farther from your destination and walking to it, or tossing a ball with a family member or pet in the backyard.

7. *Make time to unwind.* It's all right to do "nothing." You could set aside a period of time every day to relax and listen to music. You could take a warm bath. You could take a stroll around the neighborhood or find a comfortable place to practice deep breathing. You could use aromatherapy (lavender, sandalwood, clary sage,

lemon, neroli [orange blossom], bergamot). Whatever you choose, make sure it's an activity that makes you feel refreshed, renewed, and rejuvenated.

8. *Give of yourself.* Helping someone else is one of the best ways to get your mind off your own problems, but if you feel extra stressed, just use the time to *pamper yourself.* (Just be sure to pamper yourself in a health-producing way. Eating a pint of Häagen-Dazs does not qualify!)

9. *Keep a clear head* at all times. Alcohol or drugs will not cure stress. Your immune system is already suppressed by your stress—you don't need to suppress it any more by using drugs or ingesting alcohol.

10. *Pray.* Give your cares and worries to the Lord, who will carry your burdens for you.

Stress busters from nature

The following stress-busting herbs can make all the difference in your battle to rise above stress.

Siberian ginseng

Siberian ginseng is a root that belongs to the ginseng family of adaptogenic herbs. Adaptogens help build our resistance to stress. Siberian ginseng helps your body adapt to stress, and it reduces fatigue, which is often one of the underlying factors in an overstressed person's life. Ginseng improves oxygen and blood sugar metabolism as well as immune function. However, it's not advised for severe anxiety. Siberian ginseng is a stimulant, so don't take it before you go to bed or if you have high blood pressure.

Do not confuse Siberian ginseng with Panax ginseng. The Panax version can increase your body's cortisol, and cortisol is your body's stress hormone.

Valerian

Valerian is widely used in Europe as a sedative. The Chinese also use it to treat nervous conditions and insomnia. Its effect is said to be similar to benzodiazepine tranquilizers but without as many side effects. (Side effects are rare but may include headaches and stimulant effects in some people.) Valerian, like benzodiazepines, enhances the activity of GABA. Take valerian one hour before bedtime for insomnia or, in smaller amounts, two or three times a day to help relieve performance anxiety and stress. Never take valerian with alcohol. The effects of valerian use are cumulative, so you have to take it for two to three weeks before you can evaluate your results.

Passionflower

Passionflower is a climbing plant native to North America. Passionflower combined with valerian is a popular herbal remedy throughout much of Europe for insomnia, anxiety, and irritability.

St. John's wort

For twenty-four hundred years, St. John's wort has been used to treat anxiety and depression in Europe. This plant-based supplement enhances the activity of GABA. In addition, it enhances the activity of three important neurotransmitters—serotonin, norepinephrine, and dopamine. St. John's wort must be taken for at least six weeks before evaluating the results, because the effect is cumulative, not immediate. Never take St. John's wort if you are currently taking prescription antidepressants, especially one of the MAO inhibitors (Nardil, Parnate). If you stop taking a prescription antidepressant, wait at least four weeks before taking St. John's wort to make sure that no overlapping occurs. Side effects are very rare but may include dizziness and gastrointestinal irritation.

Kava

Kava comes from the root of piper methysticum, a member of the pepper tree family native to the South Pacific. Kava is proven for both short-term and long-term treatment of anxiety, tension, fear, and insomnia. Kava has a natural tranquilizing effect on the brain by acting on the amygdala, the brain's alarm center.

Never mix kava with alcohol, prescription antidepressants, benzodiazepine, tranquilizers, or sleeping pills. If you have Parkinson's disease, kava may worsen your muscular weakness. Extremely high doses of kava (ten times the normal dose) can cause vision, breathing, and muscle problems as well as yellowed or scaly skin. If kava is used properly, it can bring blessed relief from stress.

5-HTP (5-hydroxytryptophan)

The amino acid 5-HTP is derived from the seed of the griffonia tree and is related to the amino acid tryptophan. It is used to treat anxiety, insomnia, depression, and other related conditions linked with low levels of serotonin. The body uses 5-HTP to manufacture serotonin, the neurotransmitter linked to mood. By raising serotonin levels in the body, anxiety and depression can be relieved. Informal studies suggest that 5-HTP is effective for mild to moderate anxiety as well as full-blown anxiety disorders. It should be taken at the time of day when you feel the most stressed and anxious.

Stress-busting drugs vs. herbs

Which way should you go—prescription drugs or natural herbs? Ultimately you must decide for yourself, although you should always talk to your physician before discontinuing any prescription medication for stress. The following chart serves as a general guideline.

FOR MODERATE TO SEVERE ANXIETY AND CHRONIC STRESS	
PRESCRIPTION DRUGS	**HERBAL ALTERNATIVES**
Xanax	Siberian ginseng
Klonopin	Valerian
Tranxene	Kava
Valium	
Ativan	
Sleeping pills (Restoril, Dalmane, Halcion, Serax)	

FOR DEPRESSION AND ANXIETY	
PRESCRIPTION DRUGS (SSRIs)	**HERBAL ALTERNATIVES**
Paxil	St. John's wort
Zoloft	5-HTP (5-hydroxytryptophan)
Prozac	

SLEEP INDUCERS

Our minds and bodies pay the price when we shortchange ourselves on sleep. Our mood stays low along with our energy, and we are tempted to use too much caffeine or other stimulants to make up for our lack of sleep.

What we really need is simple: sleep. Often enough, our best intentions are thwarted by something as simple as eating or drinking something that produces wakefulness instead of sleep. What are some foods to avoid from dinnertime to bedtime? What are the foods that will help to promote restful sleep?

Foods to avoid before bedtime

Many foods and beverages are helpful if you want to perk up and sharpen your attention. These foods stimulate neurochemical reactions in your brain; these are *not* the foods and beverages that you want to choose in the hours before you go to bed. They are your tickets to insomnia.

Caffeine

It may go without saying, but I'll say it anyway—for several hours before bedtime (some people need to go back as far as 4:00 p.m.), avoid drinks or foods that contain caffeine. This includes coffee, tea, colas, and more. You may need to cut back on your caffeine intake during the earlier part of the day as well, or you may need to cut caffeine entirely out of your daily diet. Consult the chart of the caffeine content of various beverages (on next page) to see how much caffeine you might be taking into your body over the course of your whole day.

Caffeine is a stimulant. It activates your nervous system as well as your other major body systems. Caffeine causes your level of adrenaline to rise, which causes an increase in your heart rate, breathing rate, digestion speed (more stomach acids), and your urinary output (because of its diuretic effect). Do you want any of that to happen at bedtime? I don't think so!

Those adrenal hormones cause your liver to release stored sugar, which in turn stimulates sugar cravings to replenish the stores. This is why caffeine increases the roller-coaster effect of blood sugar swings. Right away after your morning cup of coffee, you feel energized, but later you crash.

For most people, the effects of caffeine disappear within no more than six hours, which is why coffee in the morning will not usually interfere with bedtime. Even having a caffeine-containing beverage with your lunch may not affect your sleep, but anything later than that may keep you awake. Some people are extra sensitive—they really cannot have caffeine in their systems at all. It should be a no-brainer to decide to break the caffeine habit in order to obtain the sleep your body so desperately needs.

Warning: over-the-counter cold and headache remedies may contain caffeine. Check the label or ask your pharmacist.

CAFFEINE CONTENT OF COMMON BEVERAGES	
Coffee	Brewed coffee: 60–180 mg/large cup Drip coffee: 115–150 mg/large cup Instant coffee: 30–150 mg/large cup "Decaffeinated" coffee: 3–5 mg/large cup
Tea	Brewed tea: 25–100 mg/teacup (depending on how long you leave the teabag in) Instant tea: 25–50 mg/serving Iced tea: 70 mg./12-oz. glass
Soft drinks (12-oz. can or bottle)	Jolt: 100 mg Mountain Dew: 55 mg Colas (diet or regular): 35–45 mg 7Up: 0 mg.

Alcohol

Alcohol is another stimulant you should avoid. A glass of wine may make you feel relaxed and sleepy before you go to bed, but as your body processes it, the sedative properties give way to arousing ones. This tends to jolt you awake during REM (rapid eye moment) sleep, just when you need to stay asleep.

Sugar, spicy, heavy foods

Never eat heavy (calorie- and fat-dense) foods at bedtime, especially if they are sugary (including those made of refined carbohydrates) or spicy (seasoned with hot peppers and garlic, for instance), which will especially affect you if you have a problem with heartburn. You might be able to get away with some of these foods at dinnertime, but only if your food has time to fully digest before bedtime. In other words, don't expect to sleep well if you have eaten a heavy meal at a "stylishly late" hour of eight or nine o'clock (especially if you include alcohol or after-dinner coffee with your meal).

Heavy or overlarge meals make your digestive system work too hard just when you want to settle down for the night. For some people, specific foods have this effect even when consumed in small to moderate quantities. For example, some people need to avoid beans, cucumbers, or peanuts. You can't sleep well with the discomfort of gas production and internal rumblings. You may fall asleep fast because you feel so full, but all the extra work your digestive system has to do will keep waking you up and making you sleep too lightly.

In particular, avoid meals close to bedtime that include chocolate, ham, bacon, sauerkraut, sausage, cheese, eggplant, spinach, tomatoes, sugar, and wine. These foods contain tyramine. Tyramine encourages the release of norepinephrine, which is a brain stimulant. You may also be sensitive to additives, preservatives, or agents such as MSG (monosodium glutamate), which is often found in Chinese foods. For some people, these substances have a stimulant effect.

Large or rich snacks will have the same effect as a large meal. In general, be kind to your digestive system—respect the fact that it will be moving more slowly at night.

High fluid intake

To avoid having to interrupt your sleep to urinate, limit your fluid intake in the evening hours before bedtime. It's true that you need plenty of water during your day, and it's also true that you will sleep better if you are well hydrated in general. Just try to drink most of your water earlier in the day.

High-protein foods

If you eat a high-protein snack (such as meat) before bedtime, you may feel too alert to go to sleep. Protein inhibits sleep by blocking the synthesis of serotonin.

Smoking

While not exactly a food and while seeming to have a calming effect, cigarettes and other tobacco products contain nicotine, which is a neurostimulant and which can cause sleep problems. If you are a smoker, I don't need to tell you that it would be best of all for you to stop smoking. If you are having sleep difficulties, at least you may want to try to smoke your last cigarette a few hours prior to turning in for the night.

SOME FOODS TO AVOID AT BEDTIME

All "junk food"	Meats, with the exception of turkey in small amounts
Cheese	Sauerkraut
Chocolate	Spinach
Eggplant	Sugar, desserts
Foods to which you are allergic (common allergies include dairy, wheat, and chocolate)	Tomatoes
	Wine and other alcoholic beverages
Ham, bacon, sausage	
Ice cream	

I tell my clients to avoid over-the-counter sleeping pills because of their undesirable consequences, which include lack of REM sleep (rapid eye movement, your dreaming sleep, which is essential), "hangovers," and a tendency to decrease in their effectiveness with overuse because of increased tolerance.

Foods that promote restful sleep

Now you know what *not* to eat or drink or smoke at bedtime. Are there some particular foods that can actually help you to fall asleep more quickly—and sleep "like a baby"? Yes, and the first one (for all you former babies out there) is *milk*.

Milk

Nature has it right. Milk—warm milk is especially comforting—is the traditional bedtime sleep inducer. Milk contains a certain amount of tryptophan, an amino acid that, when converted to seratonin and melatonin in the body, makes you sleepy and helps to keep you from waking up in the night. These neurotransmitters tell your nerves to slow down so your brain can slow down too.

Milk also contains calcium, which will help your brain use the tryptophan. Some people swear by a little honey in their warm milk. Sugar in large quantities will have the opposite effect, but a touch of glucose causes your brain to turn off a neurotransmitter called *orexin* that helps to keep you alert and awake. The tryptophan and calcium are not affected by warming, so you can gain the same benefits from cold milk.

Of course, if your body cannot easily digest milk or other dairy products, you should ignore this piece of advice and choose another type of food as your sleep aid.

Milk plus...

To get your brain even more calmed down, combine complex carbohydrates with milk, or choose another tryptophan-containing food altogether. What you don't want to do is eat a lot of protein *without* carbohydrates, because protein-rich foods contain the amino acid tyrosine, which will perk your brain up.

Your best choice for a bedtime snack would include both complex carbohydrates and protein, along with some calcium. Calcium will help your brain to utilize the tryptophan in your snack to manufacture melatonin. Again, if your system tolerates milk well, it does combine both tryptophan and calcium.

Eat high-protein, lower-carbohydrate meals for breakfast and lunch when you need to be at your best mentally. Then eat your dinner early enough so that it can digest before you go to bed. Meals that are high in complex carbohydrates and low to medium in protein will help you relax during the evening and make a good night's sleep easy to achieve. Eat modestly so you are not overstuffed, but be sure to eat enough so that you won't get so hungry that you eat too much for a bedtime snack. If you do need or want a bedtime snack, eat it an hour or two before you turn in for the night, in order to give the tryptophan time to work on your behalf.

For your dinner and, if required, your bedtime snack, try to choose the more sleep-inducing foods, such as the following, which is far from a complete list of options:

- Almonds, hazelnuts, peanuts
- An oatmeal-raisin cookie (with a glass of milk)
- Bananas, figs, dates, grapefruit
- Beans, if tolerated
- Brown rice
- Chili with beans, not spicy
- Eggs
- Hummus (with whole-wheat pita bread)
- Lentils
- Meats, poultry (especially turkey), seafood (modest servings)

- Milk, cottage cheese, yogurt, other low-fat dairy products
- Oats, oatmeal
- Pasta (avoid spicy sauces)
- Peanut butter or other nut butter on whole-grain bread
- Rice
- Salad with tuna chunks, sesame seeds, and whole-grain bread or crackers
- Seeds such as sunflower seeds or sesame seeds (rich in tryptophan)
- Soy milk, tofu, soybean nuts
- Tuna fish sandwich
- Whole-grain (complex carbohydrates) baked goods
- Whole-grain cereal with milk

Other sleep-promoting strategies

Maintain a bedtime routine.

People who retire and rise at the same time every day are less likely to experience insomnia or to complain about daytime fatigue.

Take a warm bath.

A hot bath (not a shower) before bedtime helps many people relax so that they can fall asleep with ease. Even if you don't take a bath, use the hour or so before you retire as a time to relax quietly.

Keep your bedroom for sleeping only.

Make sure that your bedroom is as conducive to sleep as possible. It should be a quiet, dark, peaceful place without negative associations, and it should be at a comfortable temperature for sleeping. Try to avoid having a television or a computer in your bedroom, and keep your desk and paperwork someplace else.

Skip the evening nap.

As tired as you may be, don't let yourself nod off in your easy chair. All this will do is hinder your ability to fall asleep later at your actual bedtime.

Brew a cup of chamomile tea.

If you aren't concerned about nighttime trips to the bathroom, a warm cup of golden chamomile tea might be perfect for you. It has a mildly sedating effect, and, of course, brewing it and sipping it will provide you with a built-in time of relaxation before bedtime. Use 2 or 3 heaping teaspoons of flowers per cup of boiling water and let it steep five to ten minutes.

Minimize your pain.

Sometimes you can't sleep simply because you hurt. Aches and pains can wreak havoc on your sleep. Pain dampens your strength and spirit and causes you to be discouraged and depressed. While painkillers can allow you temporary relief so you can carry on with whatever you're trying to do (including sleep), they do nothing to address the cause of the pain. In addition, painkillers can become addictive, and they can damage your stomach lining as well as your liver and kidneys.

To address pain in a natural way, start with the foods you eat. Avoid caffeine, sugar, and salty foods that create an overacidic system and cause you to retain water, which makes you feel sluggish and achy. Have a green drink each day to boost your natural defenses. Eat a vegetarian diet that is low in fats and high in minerals. Consider the following herbal pain relievers: white willow bark (a natural anti-inflammatory and analgesic), kava (a stress reliever that can help you in cases of chronic pain), valerian (a natural sedative), or St. John's wort (for nerve damage and to lift your spirits). Natural painkillers include GABA (750 mg daily), magnesium (800 mg at bedtime), and glucosamine capsules or glucosamine cream (which contains and works with your body's natural hormones to provide quick relief to inflamed joints and sore muscles caused by overwork, daily activity, or arthritis).

Try a sleep-inducing supplement.

Amino acids such as 5-HTP (5-hydroxytryptophan) act as precursors to tryptophan, which stimulates serotonin production in your brain to help alleviate anxiety. Herbs such as kava, passionflower, and valerian have been used across the world for centuries for their natural sedative qualities. Calcium and magnesium, while available in some of the suggested sleep-inducing foods such as milk and bananas, are easy to obtain in supplement form. Inositol can ensure that you will not suffer from disturbed REM (rapid eye movement) sleep.

SLEEP-INDUCING SUPPLEMENTS

Amino Acids and Hormones	5-HTP (5-hydroxytryptophan)—Take 50 mg three times a day. Enteric (coated) capsules will reduce the risk of nausea as a side effect. Melatonin—A natural hormone that promotes sound sleep DHEA (dehydroepiandrosterone)—A natural hormone that improves the quality of sleep L-theanine—An amino acid that, if taken thirty minutes before bed, promotes deep muscle relaxation
Herbs*	Kava—Kava has been used in the South Pacific for centuries for its calming properties. If using capsules, take up to 120 mg daily. Passionflower—Passionflower has a number of calming properties useful for sleep aid. If using a tincture, take twenty to thirty drops in one cup of warm water. If using capsules (500 mg), take one capsule thirty minutes before you turn out the light. Valerian—Valerian is a traditional sleep aid that has been in use for more than one thousand years. Take thirty to sixty drops in a cup of boiling water within the hour before you go to bed. If you have Valerian capsules (often standardized to 0.8 percent valeric acids), take 300 to 500 mg thirty to sixty minutes before going to bed. * Warning: Do not use herbal sleeping aids in combination with antidepressant drugs.
Minerals	Calcium—As well as helping to build healthy bones, calcium has a calming effect on the body. Take 1,500 to 2,000 mg daily in divided doses after meals and before bed. Use the chelated form of calcium to obtain the best absorption, and avoid calcium carbonate, which may contain lead. Magnesium—Magnesium should be included to aid your calcium absorption, usually in a 2:1 ratio of calcium to magnesium. Take 1,000 mg daily. You can often obtain both minerals in one supplement.

SLEEP-INDUCING SUPPLEMENTS

Vitamins	
	B-50 complex—A B-50 complex vitamin will help you cope with stress and anxiety (which keep you awake) because it will help ensure the synthesis of tryptophan to serotonin. Take one 50 mg capsule one or two times daily. (I advise against taking 100 mg capsules, because your body cannot easily absorb this amount at one time.)
	Inositol—Inositol can enhance REM sleep. Take a bedtime dose of 100 mg daily.

For more information about sleep, go to the Web site for the National Center on Sleep Disorders (a division of the National Heart, Lung, and Blood Institute Information Center), which is in Bethesda, Maryland (www.nhibi.nih.gov).

ENERGY BOOSTERS

Don't you love to feel energetic and full of life? Everything goes better when you feel that way. Sometimes, though, we sabotage ourselves when it comes to improving and sustaining our energy level all day long, especially in the category of food.

What is the best nutritional decision you can make tomorrow to ensure that you will open your front door and walk into your day with a brisk, bouncy step? That's easy—*eat breakfast.* Study after study has shown that people who eat breakfast have more energy all day long. Breakfast skippers may declare they "just don't feel like eating" first thing in the morning, but they probably overeat as the day goes on in an effort to compensate for the lack of fuel their bodies need. Skipping breakfast makes it difficult to achieve mental focus.

"Not eating breakfast basically puts your entire day in jeopardy—it's like running your car without oil and gas—using the drudge at the bottom of the gas tank," says nutrition expert Elizabeth Somer.[3]

You don't have to prepare a breakfast of bacon and eggs and pancakes. In fact, it would be a lot better if you didn't. Just eat a container of low-fat yogurt and a piece of whole-grain toast or a banana and a handful of almonds. Then proceed through the rest of your day, choosing foods that will enhance your energy, not sap it.

PROTEIN = ENERGY

Make sure to consume quality protein at every meal. This will help to give you the energy you need, and it will provide your body with slow-burning fuel throughout the day. Sources of good-quality protein include fish, lean chicken and turkey, beans, nuts, seeds, and low-fat dairy and soy products.

Protein sources contain tyrosine, the amino acid that helps produce neurotransmitters that keep you mentally alert. Tyrosine helps to build the body's natural supply of adrenaline and thyroid hormones. It is also an antioxidant and a source of quick energy, especially for the brain.

DIETARY SOURCES OF PROTEIN[4]

FOOD	SERVING	PROTEIN GRAMS
Chicken	6 ounces	85 grams
Egg	1 large	6.3 grams
Fish	6 ounces	41.2 grams
Kidney beans	½ cup	7.6 grams
Lentils	½ cup	9 grams
Skim milk	1 cup	8.4 grams
Soy milk	1 cup	6.7 grams
Tofu	½ cup	10.1 grams
Whole-wheat bread	2 slices	5.4 grams
Yogurt	8 ounces	11.9 grams

To keep yourself energized, also be sure to stay adequately hydrated. Sometimes you don't really need any food; the only boost you need is a glass or a bottle of water—really! Drink water to help both your energy and your mood improve. Be careful not to obtain your fluid intake from caffeinated beverages, even though you may be tempted to grab a cup of coffee or a cola to give yourself an energy boost. The caffeine (and sugar) will create those energy fluctuations that are so hard to deal with. The caffeine "high" is not worth the subsequent "low."

Your water requirements may vary depending on your activity level and your environment. Your home and work environment, which is likely to be heated in winter and air-conditioned in summer, may dehydrate you more quickly than you realize, especially if you live at a high altitude or in a dry climate or both.

For more even energy and mood throughout your demanding day, you might want to try eating a number of smaller meals, or modest meals interspersed with nourishing snacks, instead of the typical American three square meals a day—or skipping meals.

Nutrition for Adrenal Exhaustion

In chapter 3 ("Stress and Your Diet"), I described a problem that is all too common—adrenal exhaustion. I explained how it develops, what it feels like, and what to do about it. If you find that you are working to overcome adrenal exhaustion, remember that it requires a three-part plan of attack.

1. *Exercise.* Exercise is a huge stress reliever, and it helps bring down your high levels of cortisol while increasing endorphins and serotonin, which will inhibit the stress response. Exercise just thirty minutes a day, five times a week, and add strength training two times a week. Be sure to take breaks throughout your workday to diffuse accumulated stress. Just taking your dog for a walk will work wonders! Breathe deeply, and reflect on all of your blessings.

2. *Nutrition* is the next area you must address. Eliminate refined sugars and carbohydrates, and eat four to five servings of fruit and vegetables and three servings of whole grains daily. This will keep you energized and less apt to "stress eat." Include brown rice, almonds, garlic,

salmon, flounder, lentils, sunflower seeds, bran, brewer's yeast, and avocado in your diet.

3. The *mental* aspect of stress management is to realize that stress is not stress unless you perceive it as stress. It is how you react and act that will determine what will be detrimental to your health. Part of overcoming stress is simply recognizing that you can. With the suggestions I have outlined above, you can recover the energy you have lost and even become more energetic than you ever were before.

There is no one-size-fits-all "energy diet." To garner the benefits of feeling energized day in and day out, you need to eat a variety of foods to provide all of the amino acids (protein) you need. Avoid foods to which you are allergic or sensitive. You will need to pay attention to the requirements of your own body, some of which may change over time.

Mood Enhancers

Are you looking for the perfect "comfort food"? Do you need something that will improve your mood within minutes and maybe keep you feeling good for some time?

With all that you have learned in this book, you can figure out the perfect mood-enhancing food for your needs.

Mood food: carbs

Carbohydrates—if they are complex carbohydrates—boost your brain's serotonin levels, and serotonin is known as the "good mood" chemical. Choose whole-grain breads, brown rice, beans, and fresh vegetables instead of processed, refined carbohydrates such as white breads and white rice. Avoid carbohydrates such as candy, sweet baked goods, and junk foods, even if they are the only things available in the vending machine at work. Those are simple carbohydrates, and their sugar content alone will give you a temporary "buzz," only to let you down badly later.

Instead of playing with your blood sugar levels, keep them even by eating smart. Leave that cookie for someone else. Instead, try some air-popped popcorn, fresh fruit, or whole-grain crackers.

Mood foods that provide folic acid

Many people who suffer from low moods have been shown to have a folic-acid deficiency. If you know what to choose, you can eat foods that will supply you with extra folic acid. Choose foods such as asparagus; avocados; garbanzos, soybeans, and other beans; lentils and other legumes; oranges; broccoli; and spinach and its dark leafy cousins.

Mood foods that provide magnesium

Magnesium relaxes your tense muscles. Here again, avocados and spinach can help. You can also get magnesium from dark chocolate (in small servings, please), almonds, and pumpkin or sunflower seeds.

Mood foods that provide niacin

I mentioned niacin (also known as B_3) in chapter 5, where I described the valuable B vitamins in detail. Niacin assists in the functioning of your digestive system, and it keeps your skin and nerves healthy. It is also important for the conversion of food to energy. Some experts believe that it can help alleviate depression, anxiety, or panic. Niacin is found in dairy products, poultry, fish, lean meats, brown rice, nuts, and eggs. Legumes and breads and cereals made with enriched grains also supply some niacin. Of course, these foods also supply you with some proteins, which also give you mood-boosting energy.

Mood foods that provide zinc

If you lack zinc in your diet, you will have a very short "fuse." You will be irritable and easily angered. For your own sake and for the sake of your family and the other people around you, see if you can improve your bad mood with some zinc-containing whole-grain bread, a glass of milk, an egg or two, or even some oysters.

Mood foods are low in sodium

The average American adult consumes more than twice as much sodium in a day than is recommended. This has the negative effect of making a person retain water, which makes him or her feel sluggish. It also causes blood pressure to rise, which is hard on every part of a person's body.

Most people should be limiting their sodium intake to about 1,300 mg per day (less for older people or those with specific health concerns).

According to the Harvard Health Letter, the average adult consumes 3,000 to 4,000 mg of sodium per day.

Mood foods in moderation

Even mood-enhancing foods should not be eaten in large quantities, or you will have too much of a good thing. Don't let your low mood drive you to overeat. If you do, you will undo many of the effects of the good nutrition by raising your blood sugar and consequent insulin and cortisone levels. You want your food to *enhance* your mood, not swing it wildly back and forth.

Eat smart and healthy. Eat a well-balanced, nutritious diet that is made up mostly of an array of fresh vegetables and fruits, whole grains and nuts, healthy oils and minimal sugar, and well-chosen lean protein, and you will help both your mood and your waistline. The foods and extra supplements that you consume cannot possibly cure everything that ails you, but they definitely can improve your mood.

FEED YOUR MIND WITH POSITIVE FOOD

To be healthy in every way, you need to feed your mind more than good culinary fare and supplements. Five of the most important mood foods are as follows:

- Pray.
- Banish fear with faith.
- Fill your mind with uplifting input.
- Forgive other people.
- Love others unconditionally.

If you don't pay attention to those five elements, no amount of good nutrition can fully compensate for the state of your emotions and mind. If you don't reach up to God, who cares for you and with whom you can have a lifelong relationship through Jesus Christ, you will become self-centered and small minded. If you don't put your faith in Him, fears will rule your life. If you allow the equivalent of junk food to occupy your senses via the airwaves and the reading material you choose, your mental and emotional nutrition will take a serious nosedive. If you don't forgive other people as soon as possible for their misdeeds, intentional or accidental, and love other people with no strings attached, you will find that after a while your soul will shrivel up and your most pervasive mood will probably be one of grim resignation.

The Bible teaches us that we should not be anxious, fearful, or stressed—even about what we should eat every day—and that the solution to these troubling emotions is faith and trust in Jesus Christ. He said:

> Do not be worried about your life, as to what you will eat or what you will drink; nor for your body, as to what you will put on. Is not life more than food, and the body more than clothing? Look at the birds of the air, that they do not sow, nor reap nor gather into barns, and yet your heavenly Father feeds them. Are you not worth much more than they? And who of you by being worried can add a single hour to his life?...
>
> Do not worry then, saying, "What will we eat?" or "What will we drink?" or "What will we wear for clothing?" For the Gentiles eagerly seek all these things; for your heavenly Father knows that you need all these things.
>
> But seek first His kingdom and His righteousness, and all these things will be added to you.
>
> —Matthew 6:25–27, 31–33

God is your Father. Go to Him every day in confidence. His Word will sustain you more than any health food, vitamin, or herbal supplement. God will keep your mind and body safe.

Aim for the finest mood of all—true joy! Live the way God intended you to live. Don't blame your boss or your parents or your circumstances for your difficulties. People who have gone before you can tell you that it is possible to walk in joy even in the midst of great troubles. Always seek excellence. Do everything in your power, including changing your food intake (which includes spiritual as well as physical food), to keep yourself on the track of true joy.

FOOD SOURCES FOR SELECTED VITAMINS, MINERALS, AND OTHER NUTRIENTS

FOOD SOURCES OF CALCIUM

Food sources of calcium are ranked by milligrams of calcium per standard amount. (All are greater than 20 percent of adequate intake [AI] for adults nineteen to fifty years of age, which is 1,000 mg/day.)

FOOD, STANDARD AMOUNT	CALCIUM (MG)	CALORIES
Feta cheese, 1.5 oz.	210	113
Mozzarella cheese, whole milk, 1.5 oz.	215	128
Blue cheese, 1.5 oz.	225	150
Ricotta cheese, whole milk, ½ cup	255	214
Yogurt, plain, whole milk (8 g protein/8 oz.), 8-oz. container	275	138
Whole milk, 1 cup	276	146
Chocolate milk, 1 cup	280	208
Buttermilk, low fat, 1 cup	284	98
Reduced fat chocolate milk (2 percent), 1 cup	285	180
Two percent reduced-fat milk, 1 cup	285	122
Low-fat chocolate milk (1 percent), 1 cup	288	158
One percent low-fat milk, 1 cup	290	102
Muenster cheese, 1.5 oz.	305	156
Fat-free (skim) milk, 1 cup	306	83

FOOD, STANDARD AMOUNT	CALCIUM (MG)	CALORIES
Cheddar cheese, 1.5 oz.	307	171
Mozzarella cheese, part-skim, 1.5 oz.	311	129
Provolone cheese, 1.5 oz.	321	150
Pasteurized process American cheese food, 2 oz.	323	188
Ricotta cheese, part skim, ½ cup	335	170
Swiss cheese, 1.5 oz.	336	162
Fruit yogurt, low fat (10 g protein/8 oz.), 8-oz. Container	345	232
Plain yogurt, low-fat (12 g protein/8 oz.), 8-oz. container	415	143
Pasteurized process Swiss cheese, 2 oz.	438	190
Plain yogurt, nonfat (13 g protein/8 oz.), 8-oz. container	452	127
Romano cheese, 1.5 oz.	452	165

Nondairy Food Sources of Calcium

Nondairy food sources of calcium are ranked by milligrams of calcium per standard amount. The bioavailability may vary. Both calcium content and bioavailability should be considered when selecting dietary sources of calcium. Some plant foods have calcium that is well absorbed, but the large quantity of plant foods that would be needed to provide as much calcium as in a glass of milk may be unachievable for many. Many other calcium-fortified foods are available, but the percentage of calcium that can be absorbed is unavailable for many of them.[1]

FOOD, STANDARD AMOUNT	CALCIUM (MG)	CALORIES
Rainbow trout, farmed, cooked, 3 oz.	73	144
Dandelion greens, cooked from fresh, ½ cup	74	17

FOOD, STANDARD AMOUNT	CALCIUM (MG)	CALORIES
Clams, canned, 3 oz.	78	126
Pak-choi, Chinese cabbage, cooked from fresh, ½ cup	79	10
Beet greens, cooked from fresh, ½ cup	82	19
Blue crab, canned, 3 oz.	86	84
Okra, cooked from frozen, ½ cup	88	26
Soybeans, mature, cooked, ½ cup	88	149
Kale, cooked from frozen, ½ cup	90	20
White beans, canned, ½ cup	96	153
Cowpeas, cooked, ½ cup	106	80
Ocean perch, Atlantic, cooked, 3 oz.	116	103
Turnip greens, cooked from frozen, ½ cup	124	24
Soybeans, green, cooked, ½ cup	130	127
Spinach, cooked from frozen, ½ cup	146	30
Molasses, blackstrap, 1 Tbsp.	172	47
Collards, cooked from frozen, ½ cup	178	31
Pink salmon, canned, with bone, 3 oz.	181	118
Oatmeal, plain and flavored, instant, fortified, 1 packet prepared	99–110	97–157
Tofu, firm, prepared with nigari,* ½ cup	253	88
Sardines, Atlantic, in oil, drained, 3 oz.	325	177
Soy beverage, calcium fortified, 1 cup	368	98
Fortified ready-to-eat cereals (various), 1 oz.	236–1043	88–106

*Calcium sulfate and magnesium chloride

Food Sources of Magnesium

Food sources of magnesium are ranked by milligrams of magnesium per standard amount. (All are greater than 10 percent of RDA for adult men, which is 420 mg/day.)[2]

FOOD, STANDARD AMOUNT	MAGNESIUM (MG)	CALORIES
Brown rice, cooked, ½ cup	42	108
Haddock, cooked, 3 oz.	42	95
Buckwheat groats, roasted, cooked, ½ cup	43	78
Great northern beans, cooked, ½ cup	44	104
Oat bran, cooked, ½ cup	44	44
Oat bran muffin, 1 oz.	45	77
Cowpeas, cooked, ½ cup	46	100
Hazelnuts, 1 oz.	46	178
Okra, cooked from frozen, ½ cup	47	26
Soy beverage, 1 cup	47	127
Tofu, firm, prepared with nigari,* ½ cup	47	88
Navy beans, cooked, ½ cup	48	127
Beet greens, cooked, ½ cup	49	19
Artichokes (hearts), cooked, ½ cup	50	42
Lima beans, baby, cooked from frozen, ½ cup	50	95
Peanuts, dry roasted, 1 oz.	50	166
Soybeans, green, cooked, ½ cup	54	127
Tuna, yellowfin, cooked, 3 oz.	54	118
Oat bran, raw, ¼ cup	55	58
Bulgur, dry, ¼ cup	57	120
Black beans, cooked, ½ cup	60	114
Pollack, walleye, cooked, 3 oz.	62	96

FOOD, STANDARD AMOUNT	MAGNESIUM (MG)	CALORIES
Mixed nuts, oil roasted, with peanuts, 1 oz.	67	175
White beans, canned, ½ cup	67	154
Pine nuts, dried, 1 oz.	71	191
Cashews, dry roasted, 1 oz.	74	163
Soybeans, mature, cooked, ½ cup	74	149
Buckwheat flour, ¼ cup	75	101
Almonds, 1 oz.	78	164
Spinach, cooked from fresh, ½ cup	78	20
Spinach, canned, ½ cup	81	25
Quinoa, dry, ¼ cup	89	159
Halibut, cooked, 3 oz.	91	119
Bran ready-to-eat cereal (100 percent), ~1 oz.	103	74
Brazil nuts, 1 oz.	107	186
Pumpkin and squash seed kernels, roasted, 1 oz.	151	148

*Calcium sulfate and magnesium chloride

FOOD SOURCES OF POTASSIUM

Food sources of potassium are ranked by milligrams of potassium per standard amount. (The AI for adults is 4,700 mg/day potassium.)[3]

FOOD, STANDARD AMOUNT	POTASSIUM (MG)	CALORIES
Sweet potato, baked, 1 potato (146 g.)	694	131
Tomato paste, ¼ cup	664	54
Beet greens, cooked, ½ cup	655	19
Potato, baked, flesh, 1 potato (156 g)	610	145

FOOD, STANDARD AMOUNT	POTASSIUM (MG)	CALORIES
White beans, canned, ½ cup	595	153
Yogurt, plain, nonfat, 8-oz. container	579	127
Tomato puree, ½ cup	549	48
Clams, canned, 3 oz.	534	126
Yogurt, plain, low-fat, 8-oz. container	531	143
Prune juice, ¾ cup	530	136
Carrot juice, ¾ cup	517	71
Blackstrap molasses, 1 Tbsp.	498	47
Halibut, cooked, 3 oz.	490	119
Soybeans, green, cooked, ½ cup	485	127
Tuna, yellowfin, cooked, 3 oz.	484	118
Lima beans, cooked, ½ cup	484	104
Winter squash, cooked, ½ cup	448	40
Soybeans, mature, cooked, ½ cup	443	149
Rockfish, Pacific, cooked, 3 oz.	442	103
Cod, Pacific, cooked, 3 oz.	439	89
Bananas, 1 medium	422	105
Spinach, cooked, ½ cup	419	21
Tomato juice, ¾ cup	417	31
Tomato sauce, ½ cup	405	39
Peaches, dried, uncooked, ¼ cup	398	96
Prunes, stewed, ½ cup	398	133
Milk, nonfat, 1 cup	382	83
Pork chop, center loin, cooked, 3 oz.	382	197
Apricots, dried, uncooked, ¼ cup	378	78
Rainbow trout, farmed, cooked, 3 oz.	375	144

FOOD, STANDARD AMOUNT	POTASSIUM (MG)	CALORIES
Pork loin, center rib (roasts), lean, roasted, 3 oz.	371	190
Buttermilk, cultured, low-fat, 1 cup	370	98
Cantaloupe, ¼ medium	368	47
Milk (1–2 percent), 1 cup	366	102–122
Honeydew melon, ⅛ medium	365	58
Lentils, cooked, ½ cup	365	115
Plantains, cooked, ½ cup	358	90
Kidney beans, cooked, ½ cup	358	112
Orange juice, ¾ cup	355	85
Split peas, cooked, ½ cup	355	116
Yogurt, plain, whole milk, 8 oz. container	352	138

FOOD SOURCES OF IRON

Food sources of iron are ranked by milligrams of iron per standard amount. (All are greater than 10 percent of RDA for teen and adult females, which is 18 mg/day.)[4]

FOOD, STANDARD AMOUNT	IRON (MG)	CALORIES
Clams, canned, drained, 3 oz.	23.8	126
Fortified ready-to-eat cereals (various), ~ 1 oz.	1.8–21.1	54–127
Oysters, eastern, wild, cooked, moist heat, 3 oz.	10.2	116
Organ meats (liver, giblets), various, cooked, 3 oz.	5.2–9.9	134–235
Fortified instant cooked cereals (various), 1 packet	4.9–8.1	Varies
Soybeans, mature, cooked, ½ cup	4.4	149

FOOD, STANDARD AMOUNT	IRON (MG)	CALORIES
Pumpkin and squash seed kernels, roasted, 1 oz.	4.2	148
White beans, canned, ½ cup	3.9	153
Blackstrap molasses, 1 Tbsp.	3.5	47
Lentils, cooked, ½ cup	3.3	115
Spinach, cooked from fresh, ½ cup	3.2	21
Beef, chuck, blade roast, lean, cooked, 3 oz.	3.1	215
Beef, bottom round, lean, 0" fat, all grades, cooked, 3 oz.	2.8	182
Kidney beans, cooked, ½ cup	2.6	112
Sardines, canned in oil, drained, 3 oz.	2.5	177
Beef, rib, lean, ¼ fat, all grades, 3 oz.	2.4	195
Chickpeas, cooked, ½ cup	2.4	134
Duck, meat only, roasted, 3 oz.	2.3	171
Lamb, shoulder, arm, lean, ¼ fat, choice, cooked, 3 oz.	2.3	237
Prune juice, ¾ cup	2.3	136
Shrimp, canned, 3 oz.	2.3	102
Cowpeas, cooked, ½ cup	2.2	100
Ground beef, 15 percent fat, cooked, 3 oz.	2.2	212
Tomato puree, ½ cup	2.2	48
Lima beans, cooked, ½ cup	2.2	108
Soybeans, green, cooked, ½ cup	2.2	127
Navy beans, cooked, ½ cup	2.1	127
Refried beans, ½ cup	2.1	118

FOOD, STANDARD AMOUNT	IRON (MG)	CALORIES
Beef, top sirloin, lean, 0" fat, all grades, cooked, 3 oz.	2.0	156
Tomato paste, ¼ cup	2.0	54

SODIUM IN FOODS

Food sources of sodium are ranked by milligrams of iron per standard amount.[5]

DESCRIPTION	COMMON MEASURE	CONTENT/ MEASURE (MG)
Onion soup mix, dehydrated,	1 packet	3132
Miso	1 cup	2563
Salt, table	1 tsp.	2325
Bread crumbs, dry, seasoned	1 cup	2111
Cornmeal, self-rising, yellow	1 cup	1860
Fast-food submarine sandwich	1 sandwich, 6" roll	1651
Wheat flour, white, self-rising	1 cup	1588
Sauerkraut, canned	1 cup	1560
Fast food shrimp, breaded and fried	6–8 shrimp	1446
Potato salad, home-prepared	1 cup	1323
Tomato sauce, canned	1 cup	1284
Baking soda	1 tsp.	1259

DESCRIPTION	COMMON MEASURE	CONTENT/ MEASURE (MG)
Fast-food taco	1 large	1233
Cheese sauce, prepared from recipe	1 cup	1198
Baked beans, canned, with franks	1 cup	1114
Chicken noodle soup, canned,	1 cup	1106
Beef bouillon powder, dry	1 packet	1019
Ham, whole, roasted	3 oz.	1009
Fast-food chili with meat	1 cup	1007
Cream of chicken soup, canned	1 cup	986
Pie crust, prepared from recipe	1 pie shell	976
Fast-food corn dog	1 corn dog	973
Beef stew, canned entree	1 cup	947
Cottage cheese, low fat	1 cup	918
Crab, Alaska king, cooked, moist heat	3 oz.	911
Fast-food chimichanga, with beef	1 chimichanga	910
Soy sauce (soy plus wheat) (shoyu)	1 Tbsp.	902
White sauce, homemade, medium	1 cup	885

DESCRIPTION	COMMON MEASURE	CONTENT/ MEASURE (MG)
Kidney beans, canned	1 cup	873
Chicken pot pie, frozen	1 small pie	857
Corned beef, canned	3 oz.	856
Onion soup, dehydrated, prepared	1 cup	849
Dill pickles	1 pickle	833
Tuna fish salad	1 cup	824
Hamburger, large, plus condiments	1 sandwich	824
Vegetable soup, canned	1 cup	822
Pie crust, frozen, baked	1 pie shell	815
Pretzels, hard, plain, salted	10 pretzels	814
Dried beef	1 oz.	791
Turkey and gravy, frozen	5-oz. package	787
Fast-food taco salad	1½ cups	762
Refried beans, canned	1 cup	753
Tomato soup, canned, with milk	1 cup	744
Herring, Atlantic, pickled	3 oz.	740
Bacon, Canadian, grilled	2 slices	719
Chickpeas (garbanzos), canned	1 cup	718

DESCRIPTION	COMMON MEASURE	CONTENT/ MEASURE (MG)
Crab, imitation, (from surimi)	3 oz.	715
Chicken, canned, meat only	5 oz.	714
Teriyaki sauce, ready to serve	1 Tbsp.	690
Fast-food hot dog, plain	1 sandwich	670
Fast-food pizza, pepperoni	1 slice 14" pie	670
Salmon, smoked	3 oz.	667
Mushrooms, canned, drained	1 cup	663
Shrimp, canned	3 oz.	661
Braunschweiger (liver sausage)	2 slices	658
Tomato juice, canned, with salt	1 cup	654
Vegetable juice cocktail, canned	1 cup	653
Ham, sliced, extra lean	2 slices	627
Frankfurter, chicken	1 frank	617
Salami, cooked, beef and pork	2 slices	604
Biscuit, prepared from recipe	4" biscuit	586
Tomatoes, canned, stewed	1 cup	564
Bread stuffing, dry mix, prepared	½ cup	543
Graham crackers	1 cup	508

DESCRIPTION	COMMON MEASURE	CONTENT/ MEASURE (MG)
Frankfurter, beef and pork	1 frank	504
Croutons, seasoned	1 cup	495
Baking powder, double acting	1 tsp.	488
Salmon, pink, canned	3 oz.	471
Bagel, egg	4" bagel	449
Bacon, cooked	3 medium slices	439
Beef jerky	1 large piece	438
Jalapeno peppers, canned	¼ cup	434
Green peas, canned	1 cup	428
Croissant, butter	1 croissant	424
Bologna, beef and pork	2 slices	417
Blue cheese	1 oz.	395
Milk, canned, condensed, sweetened	1 cup	389
Kellogg's Raisin Bran cereal	1 cup	362
American cheese	1 oz.	359–422
Turkey gravy, canned	¼ cup	344
Milk shake, thick chocolate	10.6 fl. oz.	333
Danish pastry, fruit	1 pastry	333
Pita bread, white	6½" pita	322
Tuna fish, canned in water	3 oz.	320

DESCRIPTION	COMMON MEASURE	CONTENT/ MEASURE (MG)
Cheese, camembert	1 wedge	320
Cheese, feta	1 oz.	316
Kellogg's Rice Krispies cereal	1¼ cups	314
Rolls, hard (includes kaiser)	1 roll	310
Cheese, ricotta, part-skim milk	1 cup	308
Tomatoes, canned, whole	1 cup	307
Tuna fish, light, canned in oil	3 oz.	301
Tuna fish, light, canned in water	3 oz.	287
Tortilla chips, nacho flavor, low fat	1 oz.	284
Milk, canned, evaporated	1 cup	267
Sauce, hoisin, ready to serve	1 Tbsp.	258
Milk, buttermilk, low fat	1 cup	257
Tomato paste, canned, no salt added	1 cup	257
Doughnuts, cake type, plain	1 medium	257
Cheese, provolone	1 oz.	248
English muffin, plain, toasted,	1 muffin	248
Salad dressing, Italian, commercial	1 Tbsp.	243
Muffin, oat bran	1 muffin	224

Appendix A

DESCRIPTION	COMMON MEASURE	CONTENT/ MEASURE (MG)
Bread, pumpernickel	1 slice	215
Chocolate cake, chocolate frosting	1 piece	214
General Mills Cheerios cereal	1 cup	213
Potato chips, barbecue flavor	1 oz.	213
Bread, rye	1 slice	211
Pork/beef sausage, fresh, cooked	2 links	209
Rolls, hamburger or hot dog, plain	1 roll	206
Kellogg's Corn Flakes cereal	1 cup	202
Pork sausage, fresh, cooked	1 patty	202
Chinese noodles, chow mein	1 cup	198
Olives, ripe, canned	5 large	192
Spinach, frozen, cooked, no salt	1 cup	184
Muenster cheese	1 oz.	178
Mozzarella cheese, whole milk	1 oz.	178
Cheddar cheese	1 oz.	176
Yogurt, plain, skim milk	8-oz. container	175
Ketchup	1 Tbsp.	167
Melba toast, plain	4 pieces	166

DESCRIPTION	COMMON MEASURE	CONTENT/ MEASURE (MG)
Pita bread, white	4" pita	150
Bread, whole wheat, commercial	1 slice	148
Molasses cookie	1 cookie, large (3½" to 4")	147
Mars Milky Way candy bar	1 bar (2.15 oz)	146
Rolls, dinner, plain, commercial	1 roll	146
Salad dressing, Russian	1 Tbsp.	144
Cocoa mix, powder	3 heaping tsp.	143
Soy milk	1 cup	135
Margarine, regular, salt added	1 Tbsp.	133
Bread, whole wheat	1 slice	133
Sunflower seeds, dry roasted, salted	¼ cup	131
Saltine crackers	4 crackers	129
Barbecue sauce	1 Tbsp.	128
Swordfish, cooked, dry heat	1 piece	122–131
Pickle relish, sweet	1 Tbsp.	122
Oriental mix snack, rice based	1 oz. (about ¼ cup)	117
Artichokes, boiled, no salt added	1 medium	114

DESCRIPTION	COMMON MEASURE	CONTENT/ MEASURE (MG)
Neufchatel cheese	1 oz.	113
Egg substitute, liquid	¼ cup	111
Crackers, whole wheat	4 crackers	105
Milk, nonfat	1 cup	103
Salsa, ready to serve	1 Tbsp.	96
Crackers, rye, plain	1 wafer	87
Rice beverage, Rice Dream, canned	1 cup	86
Granola bars, hard, plain	1 bar	83
Butter, salted	1 Tbsp.	82
Egg, whole, raw, fresh	1 extra large	81
Oat cereal, instant, plain	1 packet	80
Parmesan cheese, grated	1 Tbsp.	76
Peanut butter, smooth, with salt	1 Tbsp.	73
Carrot juice, canned	1 cup	68
Turkey, dark meat, roasted	3 oz.	66
Turkey, light meat, roasted	3 oz.	54
Hummus, commercial	1 Tbsp.	53
Ice cream, vanilla	½ cup	53

DESCRIPTION	COMMON MEASURE	CONTENT/ MEASURE (MG)
Beef, top sirloin, trimmed to ⅛" fat	3 oz.	52
Lemon juice, canned/bottled	1 cup	51
Cornmeal, whole grain, yellow	1 cup	43
Tomatoes, sun dried	1 piece	42
Pork, fresh, loin, bone in, cooked	3 oz.	40
Lime juice, canned/bottled	1 cup	39
Broccoli, raw	1 cup	29
Melons, honeydew, raw	⅛ melon	29
Tortillas, ready to bake or fry, corn	1 tortilla	12
Seaweed, spirulina, dried	1 Tbsp.	10
Tofu, firm (nigari)	¼ block	10
Bulgur, cooked	1 cup	9
Tomatoes, raw	1 cup	9
Baking chocolate, unsweetened	1 square	7
Potatoes, without skin, without salt	1 potato	7
Buckwheat groats, roasted	1 cup	7
Cream substitute, powdered	1 tsp.	4
Mushrooms, raw	1 cup	4

DESCRIPTION	COMMON MEASURE	CONTENT/ MEASURE (MG)
Cereals, ready to eat, puffed	1 cup	0
Lemon juice, raw	juice of 1 lemon	0
Apricots, raw	1 apricot	0
Nuts, almonds	1 oz. (24 nuts)	0
Oil, cooking, all types	1 Tbsp.	0
Grapefruit, raw, white, all areas	½ grapefruit	0
Nectarine, raw	1 nectarine	0
Orange, raw	1 orange	0
Peach, raw	1 peach	0
Plum, raw	1 plum	0
Pear, raw	1 pear	0

FOOD SOURCES OF VITAMIN C

Food sources of vitamin C are ranked by milligrams of vitamin C per standard amount. (All provide greater than 20 percent of RDA for adult men, which is 90 mg/day.)[6]

FOOD, STANDARD AMOUNT	VITAMIN C (MG)	CALORIES
Guava, raw, ½ cup	188	56
Red sweet pepper, raw, ½ cup	142	20
Red sweet pepper, cooked, ½ cup	116	19
Kiwi fruit, 1 medium	70	46
Orange, raw, 1 medium	70	62
Orange juice, ¾ cup	61–93	79–84
Green pepper, sweet, raw, ½ cup	60	15

FOOD, STANDARD AMOUNT	VITAMIN C (MG)	CALORIES
Green pepper, sweet, cooked, ½ cup	51	19
Grapefruit juice, ¾ cup	50–70	71–86
Vegetable juice cocktail, ¾ cup	50	34
Strawberries, raw, ½ cup	49	27
Brussels sprouts, cooked, ½ cup	48	28
Cantaloupe, ¼ medium	47	51
Papaya, raw, ¼ medium	47	30
Kohlrabi, cooked, ½ cup	45	24
Broccoli, raw, ½ cup	39	15
Edible pod peas, cooked, ½ cup	38	34
Broccoli, cooked, ½ cup	37	26
Sweet potato, canned, ½ cup	34	116
Tomato juice, ¾ cup	33	31
Cauliflower, cooked, ½ cup	28	17
Pineapple, raw, ½ cup	28	37
Kale, cooked, ½ cup	27	18
Mango, ½ cup	23	54

FOOD SOURCES OF VITAMIN A

Food sources of vitamin A are ranked by micrograms Retinol Activity Equivalents (RAE) of vitamin A per standard amount.[7]

FOOD, STANDARD AMOUNT	VITAMIN A (MCG RAE)	CALORIES
Organ meats (liver, giblets), various, cooked, 3 oz.	1490–9126	134–235
Carrot juice, ¾ cup	1692	71
Sweet potato with peel, baked, 1 medium	1096	103
Pumpkin, canned, ½ cup	953	42

FOOD, STANDARD AMOUNT	VITAMIN A (MCG RAE)	CALORIES
Carrots, cooked from fresh, ½ cup	671	27
Spinach, cooked from frozen, ½ cup	573	30
Collards, cooked from frozen, ½ cup	489	31
Kale, cooked from frozen, ½ cup	478	20
Mixed vegetables, canned, ½ cup	474	40
Turnip greens, cooked from frozen, ½ cup	441	24
Instant cooked cereals, fortified, prepared, 1 packet	285–376	75–97
Various ready-to-eat cereals, with added vit. A, ~1 oz.	180–376	100–117
Carrot, raw, 1 small	301	20
Beet greens, cooked, ½ cup	276	19
Winter squash, cooked, ½ cup	268	38
Dandelion greens, cooked, ½ cup	260	18
Cantaloupe, raw, ¼ medium melon	233	46
Mustard greens, cooked, ½ cup	221	11
Pickled herring, 3 oz.	219	222
Red sweet pepper, cooked, ½ cup	186	19
Chinese cabbage, cooked, ½ cup	180	10

FOOD SOURCES OF VITAMIN E

Food sources of vitamin E are ranked by milligrams of vitamin E per standard amount. (All provide greater than 10 percent of RDA for vitamin E for adults, which is 15 mg a-tocopherol [AT]/day.)[8]

FOOD, STANDARD AMOUNT	AT (MG)	CALORIES
Fortified ready-to-eat cereals, ~1 oz.	1.6–12.8	90–107
Sunflower seeds, dry roasted, 1 oz.	7.4	165
Almonds, 1 oz.	7.3	164
Sunflower oil, high linoleic, 1 Tbsp.	5.6	120
Cottonseed oil, 1 Tbsp.	4.8	120
Safflower oil, high oleic, 1 Tbsp.	4.6	120
Hazelnuts (filberts), 1 oz.	4.3	178
Mixed nuts, dry roasted, 1 oz.	3.1	168
Turnip greens, frozen, cooked, ½ cup	2.9	24
Tomato paste, ¼ cup	2.8	54
Pine nuts, 1 oz.	2.6	191
Peanut butter, 2 Tbsp.	2.5	192
Tomato puree, ½ cup	2.5	48
Tomato sauce, ½ cup	2.5	39
Canola oil, 1 Tbsp.	2.4	124
Wheat germ, toasted, plain, 2 Tbsp.	2.3	54
Peanuts, 1 oz.	2.2	166
Avocado, raw, ½ avocado	2.1	161
Carrot juice, canned, ¾ cup	2.1	71
Peanut oil, 1 Tbsp.	2.1	119
Corn oil, 1 Tbsp.	1.9	120
Olive oil, 1 Tbsp.	1.9	119
Spinach, cooked, ½ cup	1.9	21
Dandelion greens, cooked, ½ cup	1.8	18
Sardine, Atlantic, in oil, drained, 3 oz.	1.7	177
Blue crab, cooked/canned, 3 oz.	1.6	84

FOOD, STANDARD AMOUNT	AT (MG)	CALORIES
Brazil nuts, 1 oz.	1.6	186
Herring, Atlantic, pickled, 3 oz.	1.5	222

CARBOHYDRATE CONTENT OF SELECTED FOODS

Food sources of carbohydrate are ranked by grams per standard amount.[9]

DESCRIPTION	COMMON MEASURE	CONTENT/ MEASURE (G)
Raisins, seedless	1 cup	114.81
Cornmeal, degermed, yellow	1 cup	107.20
Semisweet chocolate pieces	1 cup	106.01
Wheat flour, white, bleached	1 cup	95.39
Cornmeal, whole grain, yellow	1 cup	93.81
Snacks, trail mix, tropical	1 cup	91.84
Wheat flour, whole grain	1 cup	87.08
Chocolate shake, fast food	16 fl. oz.	68.27
Oat bran, raw	1 cup	62.25
Beans, white, canned	1 cup	57.48
Plantains, raw	1 medium	57.08
Chickpeas (garbanzos), canned	1 cup	54.29
Baked beans, canned, plain	1 cup	53.70
Tomato paste	1 cup	49.54
Bagels, egg	4" bagel	47.17
Kellogg's Raisin Bran	1 cup	46.54

DESCRIPTION	COMMON MEASURE	CONTENT/ MEASURE (G)
Carbonated beverage, orange	12 fl. oz.	45.76
Danish pastry, fruit	1 pastry	45.06
Biscuits, plain or buttermilk	4" biscuit	45.05
Bagels, plain	4" bagel	44.95
Beans, pinto, boiled	1 cup	44.84
Brown rice, long grain, cooked	1 cup	44.77
White rice, long grain, cooked	1 cup	44.51
Mars Milky Way candy bar	1 bar (2.15 oz.)	43.74
Yogurt, fruit, low fat	8-oz. container	43.24
Spaghetti, cooked	1 cup	43.20
Macaroni, cooked	1 cup	43.20
Potato, baked, flesh and skin	1 potato	42.72
General Mills Basic 4 cereal	1 cup	42.35
Carbonated beverage, grape soda	12 fl. oz.	41.66
Peas, split, boiled	1 cup	41.36
General Mills Total Raisin Bran	1 cup	41.25
Mandarin oranges, light syrup	1 cup	40.80
Beans, black, boiled	1 cup	40.78
Marshmallows	1 cup	40.65
Quaker low-fat Granola, raisins	½ cup	40.59
Noodles, egg, cooked	1 cup	40.26
Beans, kidney, red, canned	1 cup	39.91
Lentils, boiled	1 cup	39.86

DESCRIPTION	COMMON MEASURE	CONTENT/ MEASURE (G)
Carbonated beverage, root beer	12 fl. oz.	39.22
Refried beans, canned	1 cup	39.14
Pineapple, canned, juice pack	1 cup	39.09
Noodles, egg, spinach, cooked	1 cup	38.80
Spaghetti, whole wheat, cooked	1 cup	37.16
Toaster pastries, fruit	1 pastry	36.97
Snickers candy bar	1 bar (2 oz.)	36.83
Potatoes, mashed with whole milk	1 cup	36.81
Couscous, cooked	1 cup	36.46
Shredded wheat cereal, plain	2 biscuits	36.23
Cake, yellow, commercial, frosted	1 piece	35.46
Carbonated beverage, cola	12 fl. oz.	35.37
Mangos, raw	1 mango	35.19
Wild rice, cooked	1 cup	35.00
Eggnog	1 cup	34.39
Cranberry juice cocktail, bottled	8 fl. oz.	34.21
Popcorn, caramel coated, peanuts	1 cup	33.89
Bulgur, cooked	1 cup	33.82
Buckwheat groats, roasted, cooked	1 cup	33.50
Pita bread, white,	6½" pita	33.42
Lima beans, ford hook, boiled	1 cup	32.84
Corn, sweet, yellow, boiled	1 cup	31.65

DESCRIPTION	COMMON MEASURE	CONTENT/ MEASURE (G)
Shortcake, prepared from recipe	1 shortcake	31.53
Onion rings, fast food, breaded/fried	8–9 rings	31.32
Cereals, corn grits, white	1 cup	31.15
Cereals, corn grits, yellow	1 cup	31.15
Dates, deglet noor	5 dates	31.14
Sweet rolls, cinnamon, raisins	1 roll	30.54
Rolls, hard (includes kaiser)	1 roll	30.04
Papayas, raw	1 papaya	29.82
Angel food cake, dry mix, prepared	1 piece	29.35
Milk, canned, evaporated, nonfat	1 cup	29.06
Apple juice, unsweetened	1 cup	28.97
Kellogg's Rice Krispies	1¼ cup	28.22
Sauce, spaghetti/ marinara	1 cup	28.18
Cream of Wheat cereal, regular	1 cup	27.61
Applesauce, canned, unsweetened	1 cup	27.55
Muffin, oat bran	1 muffin	27.53
English muffins, plain, toasted,	1 muffin	27.38
KIT KAT wafer candy bar	1 bar (1.5 oz)	27.13
Kellogg's Nutri-Grain cereal bar	1 bar	26.97
Banana, raw	1 banana	26.95
Orange juice, from concentrate	1 cup	26.84

DESCRIPTION	COMMON MEASURE	CONTENT/ MEASURE (G)
Plums, dried (prunes), uncooked	5 prunes	26.83
General Mills Rice Chex cereal	1¼ cup	26.6
Cheeseburger, fast food, regular	1 sandwich	26.53
Jelly beans	10 large	26.52
Danish pastry, cheese	1 danish	26.41
Croissant, butter	1 croissant	26.11
Milk, chocolate, low fat	1 cup	26.10
Puddings, chocolate, ready to eat	4 oz.	25.99
Noodles, Chinese, chow mein	1 cup	25.89
Milk, chocolate, whole	1 cup	25.85
General Mills Kix cereal	1⅓ cup	25.80
General Mills Corn Chex cereal	1 cup	25.80
Frosting, vanilla, creamy, prepared	¹⁄₁₂ package	25.80
Orange juice, raw	1 cup	25.79
Pears, raw	1 pear	25.66
Milk, canned, evaporated	1 cup	25.30
Oat bran, cooked	1 cup	25.05
Reese's Peanut Butter Cups	1 package (contains 2)	24.91
Kellogg's Product 19 cereal	1 cup	24.90
Rice Dream beverage, canned	1 cup	24.84
Kellogg's Corn Flakes cereal	1 cup	24.39
Alcoholic liqueur, coffee, 53 proof	1.5 fl oz.	24.34

DESCRIPTION	COMMON MEASURE	CONTENT/ MEASURE (G)
General Mills Wheaties cereal	1 cup	24.30
General Mills Wheat Chex cereal	1 cup	24.30
Doughnuts, cake type, plain	1 medium	23.36
Peas, green, frozen, cooked, boiled, drained, without salt	1 cup	22.82
Grapefruit juice, white, raw	1 cup	22.72
Sherbet, orange	½ cup	22.50
Kellogg's All-Bran cereal	½ cup	22.27
General Mills Cheerios cereal	1 cup	22.20
Kellogg's Special K cereal	1 cup	22.01
Watermelon, raw	1 wedge	21.59
Blueberries, raw	1 cup	21.01
Soybeans, green, boiled, drained	1 cup	19.89
Granola bar, soft, chocolate chip	1 bar	19.59
Pineapple, raw, all varieties	1 cup	19.58
Fish, tuna salad	1 cup	19.29
Apples, raw, with skin	1 apple	19.06
Soup, vegetable, canned	1 cup	19.01
Miso	1 cup	18.20
Squash, winter, all varieties, baked	1 cup	18.14
Tomato sauce, canned	1 cup	18.06
Yogurt, plain, skim milk	8-oz. container	17.43
Honey	1 Tbsp.	17.30

DESCRIPTION	COMMON MEASURE	CONTENT/ MEASURE (G)
Cookies, oatmeal, commercial	1 cookie, regular	17.18
Pound cake, commercial, fat free	1 slice	17.08
Soybeans, boiled,	1 cup	17.08
Soup, chicken noodle, canned	1 cup	17.04
Ice cream, vanilla, light	½ cup	17.03
Instant oat cereal, plain	1 packet	16.97
Beets, boiled, drained	1 cup	16.93
Ice cream, vanilla, rich	½ cup	16.49
Onions, raw	1 cup	16.18
Lettuce, iceberg	1 head	16.01
Carob candies	1 oz.	15.96
Lemon juice, canned or bottled	1 cup	15.81
Tomatoes, canned, stewed	1 cup	15.78
Crackers, melba toast, plain	4 pieces	15.32
Bread, pumpernickel	1 slice	15.20
Bread, pumpernickel, toasted	1 slice	15.14
Potato chips, plain, unsalted	1 oz.	15.00
Cream of chicken soup, milk	1 cup	14.98
Raspberries, raw	1 cup	14.69
Oriental mix snacks, rice based	1 oz. (about ¼ cup)	14.63
Melons, honeydew, raw	⅛ melon	14.54
Potato chips, dried potatoes, plain	1 oz.	14.46
Nectarine, raw	1 nectarine	14.35
Pancakes, plain, frozen,	1 pancake	14.14

DESCRIPTION	COMMON MEASURE	CONTENT/ MEASURE (G)
Rolls, dinner, plain,	1 roll	14.11
Blackberries, raw	1 cup	13.84
Jams and preserves	1 Tbsp.	13.77
Maple syrup	1 Tbsp.	13.42
Artichokes, boiled, drained	1 medium	13.42
Jellies	1 Tbsp.	13.29
Grapefruit, raw, all types	½ grapefruit	13.11
Cheese, ricotta, part-skim milk	1 cup	12.64
Beer, regular, all types	12 fl. oz.	12.60
Soy milk, fluid	1 cup	12.08
Milk, reduced fat, 2 percent milk fat	1 cup	11.42
Fig bar cookie	1 cookie	11.34
Kiwi fruit, raw	1 medium	11.14
Molasses cookie	1 cookie, medium	11.07
Kohlrabi, boiled, drained	1 cup	11.04
Milk, whole, 3.25 percent milk fat	1 cup	11.03
Vegetable juice cocktail, canned	1 cup	11.01
Pancakes, plain, dry mix, prepared	1 pancake	10.98
Crackers, whole wheat	4 crackers	10.98
Cucumber, with peel, raw	1 large	10.93
Cherries, sweet, raw	10 cherries	10.89
Cookie, vanilla sandwich	1 cookie	10.82
Graham crackers, plain or honey	2 squares	10.75
Sauerkraut, canned	1 cup	10.10

DESCRIPTION	COMMON MEASURE	CONTENT/ MEASURE (G)
Spinach, boiled, drained	1 cup	9.80
Peach, raw	1 peach	9.35
Collards, boiled, drained	1 cup	9.33
Cream of chicken soup, water	1 cup	9.27
Crackers, rye, wafers, plain	1 wafer	8.84
Peanut butter cookie, commercial	1 cookie, regular	8.84
Beans, snap, green, boiled, drained	1 cup	8.71
Crackers, saltines	4 crackers	8.51
Baking chocolate, unsweetened	1 square	8.46
Sugar cookie, homemade	1 cookie	8.40
Taco shells, baked	1 medium	8.30
Squash, summer, all types, boiled	1 cup	7.76
Sunflower seeds, dry roasted	¼ cup	7.70
Pistachio nuts, dry roasted	1 oz. (47 nuts)	7.59
Plum, raw	1 plum	7.54
Carrot, raw	1 carrot	6.90
Popcorn, air popped	1 cup	6.22
Peanuts, all types, dry roasted	1 oz. (approx 28)	6.10
Crackers, cheese, regular	10 crackers	5.82
Cheese, cottage, creamed	1 cup	5.63
Almonds	1 oz. (24 nuts)	5.60
Peppers, sweet, green, raw	1 pepper	5.52

DESCRIPTION	COMMON MEASURE	CONTENT/ MEASURE (G)
Cauliflower, raw	1 cup	5.30
Pickle relish, sweet	1 Tbsp.	5.26
Mung beans, sprouted, boiled	1 cup	5.20
Crackers, wheat, regular	4 crackers	5.19
Shrimp, breaded and fried	6 large	5.16
Tomatoes, red, ripe, raw	1 tomato	4.82
Peanut butter, smooth	1 Tbsp.	3.13
Hard candy	1 small piece	2.94
Cocoa, dry powder, unsweetened	1 Tbsp.	2.93
Sauce, teriyaki, ready to serve	1 Tbsp.	2.87
Tofu, soft (nigari)	1 piece	2.16
Hummus, commercial	1 Tbsp.	2.00
Salsa, ready to serve	1 Tbsp.	1.00
Garlic, raw	1 clove	0.99
Egg, whole, raw, fresh	1 extra large	0.45
Fish, all types	all portion sizes	0.00
Beef, all types	all portion sizes	0.00
Pork, all types	all portion sizes	0.00
Lamb, all types	all portion sizes	0.00
Poultry, all types	all portion sizes	0.00
Oil, all types	all portion sizes	0.00
Carbonated beverage, low calorie	12 fl. oz.	0.00
Water	8 fl. oz	0.00
Coffee, all types	all portion sizes	0.00

FOOD SOURCES OF DIETARY FIBER

Food sources of dietary fiber are ranked by grams of dietary fiber per standard amount. (All are greater than 10 percent of AI for adult women, which is 25 g/day.)[10]

FOOD, STANDARD AMOUNT	DIETARY FIBER (G)	CALORIES
Navy beans, cooked, ½ cup	9.5	128
Bran ready-to-eat cereal (100 percent), ½ cup	8.8	78
Kidney beans, canned, ½ cup	8.2	109
Split peas, cooked, ½ cup	8.1	116
Lentils, cooked, ½ cup	7.8	115
Black beans, cooked, ½ cup	7.5	114
Pinto beans, cooked, ½ cup	7.7	122
Lima beans, cooked, ½ cup	6.6	108
Artichoke, globe, cooked, 1 each	6.5	60
White beans, canned, ½ cup	6.3	154
Chickpeas, cooked, ½ cup	6.2	135
Great northern beans, cooked, ½ cup	6.2	105
Cowpeas, cooked, ½ cup	5.6	100
Soybeans, mature, cooked, ½ cup	5.2	149
Bran ready-to-eat cereals, various, ~1 oz.	2.6–5.0	90–108
Crackers, rye wafers, plain, 2 wafers	5.0	74
Sweet potato, baked, with peel, 1 medium (146 g.)	4.8	131
Asian pear, raw, 1 small	4.4	51
Green peas, cooked, ½ cup	4.4	67
Whole-wheat English muffin, 1 each	4.4	134
Pear, raw, 1 small	4.3	81
Bulgur, cooked, ½ cup	4.1	76
Mixed vegetables, cooked, ½ cup	4.0	59

FOOD, STANDARD AMOUNT	DIETARY FIBER (G)	CALORIES
Raspberries, raw, ½ cup	4.0	32
Sweet potato, boiled, no peel, 1 medium (156 g.)	3.9	119
Blackberries, raw, ½ cup	3.8	31
Potato, baked, with skin, 1 medium	3.8	161
Soybeans, green, cooked, ½ cup	3.8	127
Stewed prunes, ½ cup	3.8	133
Figs, dried, ¼ cup	3.7	93
Dates, ¼ cup	3.6	126
Oat bran, raw, ¼ cup	3.6	58
Pumpkin, canned, ½ cup	3.6	42
Spinach, frozen, cooked, ½ cup	3.5	30
Shredded wheat ready-to-eat cereals, various, ~1 oz.	2.8–3.4	96
Almonds, 1 oz.	3.3	164
Apple with skin, raw, 1 medium	3.3	72
Brussels sprouts, frozen, cooked, ½ cup	3.2	33
Whole-wheat spaghetti, cooked, ½ cup	3.1	87
Banana, 1 medium	3.1	105
Orange, raw, 1 medium	3.1	62
Oat bran muffin, 1 small	3.0	178
Guava, 1 medium	3.0	37
Pearled barley, cooked, ½ cup	3.0	97
Sauerkraut, canned, solids, and liquids, ½ cup	3.0	23
Tomato paste, ¼ cup	2.9	54
Winter squash, cooked, ½ cup	2.9	38
Broccoli, cooked, ½ cup	2.8	26
Parsnips, cooked, chopped, ½ cup	2.8	55
Turnip greens, cooked, ½ cup	2.5	15
Collards, cooked, ½ cup	2.7	25

FOOD, STANDARD AMOUNT	DIETARY FIBER (G)	CALORIES
Okra, frozen, cooked, ½ cup	2.6	26
Peas, edible-podded, cooked, ½ cup	2.5	42

DIETARY SOURCES OF PROTEIN

Food sources of protein are ranked by grams of protein per standard amount.[11]

FOOD	SERVING	WEIGHT IN GRAMS	PROTEIN GRAMS	% DAILY VALUE
Hamburger, extra lean	6 oz.	170	48.6	97
Chicken, roasted	6 oz.	170	42.5	85
Fish	6 oz.	170	41.2	82
Tuna, water packed	6 oz.	170	40.1	80
Beefsteak, broiled	6 oz.	170	38.6	77
Cottage cheese	1 cup	225	28.1	56
Cheese pizza	2 slices	128	15.4	31
Yogurt, low fat	8 oz.	227	11.9	24
Tofu	½ cup	126	10.1	20
Lentils, cooked	½ cup	99	9	18
Skim milk	1 cup	245	8.4	17
Split peas, cooked	½ cup	98	8.1	16
Whole milk	1 cup	244	8	16
Lentil soup	1 cup	242	7.8	16

FOOD	SERVING	WEIGHT IN GRAMS	PROTEIN GRAMS	% DAILY VALUE
Kidney beans, cooked	½ cup	87	7.6	15
Cheddar cheese	1 oz.	28	7.1	14
Macaroni, cooked	1 cup	140	6.8	14
Soy milk	1 cup	245	6.7	13
Egg	1 large	50	6.3	13
Whole-wheat bread	2 slices	56	5.4	11
White bread	2 slices	60	4.9	10
Rice, cooked	1 cup	158	4.3	9
Broccoli, cooked	5" piece	140	4.2	8
Baked potato	2x5 inches	156	3	6
Corn, cooked	1 ear	77	2.6	5

SUGARS IN SELECTED FOODS

Food sources of sugar are ranked by grams of sugar per standard amount.[12]

DESCRIPTION	MEASURE	CONTENT/MEASURE (G)
Milk, condensed, sweetened	1 cup	166.46
Grape juice concentrate	6 fl. oz.	95.19
Chocolate bits, semisweet	1 cup	91.56
Raisins, seedless	1 cup	85.83

DESCRIPTION	MEASURE	CONTENT/MEASURE (G)
Orange juice concentrate	6 fl. oz.	79.60
Peaches, frozen, sweetened	1 cup	55.45
Yogurt, fruit, low fat	8-oz. container	43.24
Applesauce, canned, sweetened	1 cup	42.08
Carbonated root beer	12 fl. oz.	39.22
Mandarin oranges, canned	1 cup	39.03
Grape juice, bottled, unsweetened	1 cup	37.60
Milky Way candy bar	1 bar (2.15 oz.)	37.00
Pineapple, juice pack	1 cup	35.98
Carbonated cola, with caffeine	12 fl. oz.	33.19
Carbonated Sprite, no caffeine	12 fl. oz.	33.05
Carbonated ginger ale	12 fl. oz.	31.84
Mangos, raw	1 mango	30.64
Cranberry juice cocktail, bottled	8 fl. oz.	30.03
Milk, canned, evaporated, nonfat	1 cup	29.06
Marshmallows	1 cup	28.78

DESCRIPTION	MEASURE	CONTENT/MEASURE (G)
Snickers candy bar	1 bar (2 oz.)	28.43
Tomato paste, canned	1 cup	27.27
Apple juice, unsweetened	1 cup	27.03
Plantains, raw	1 medium	26.85
Dates, deglet noor	5 dates	26.29
Cake, white, no frosting	1 piece	26.26
Graham crackers, all types	1 cup	26.12
Peaches, canned, juice pack	1 cup	25.47
Milk, canned, evaporated	1 cup	25.30
Applesauce, unsweetened	1 cup	24.62
Frosting, vanilla, ready to eat	1/12 package	23.98
Baked beans, canned	1 cup	22.96
Pudding, vanilla, ready to eat	4 oz.	22.83
Milk chocolate candy bar	1 bar (1.55 oz.)	22.66
Pasta sauce, marinara, ready to serve	1 cup	22.20
Reese's Peanut Butter Cups	1 package (contains 2)	21.23
Orange juice, raw	1 cup	20.83

DESCRIPTION	MEASURE	CONTENT/MEASURE (G)
Cocoa mix, powder	3 heaping tsp.	20.50
KIT KAT wafer bar	1 bar (1.5 oz.)	20.45
Pudding, chocolate, ready to eat	4 oz.	20.17
Jelly beans	10 large	19.85
Toaster pastries, chocolate fudge	1 pastry	19.76
Danish pastry, fruit	1 danish	19.55
Cereal, Kellogg's Raisin Bran	1 cup	19.52
Sherbet, orange	½ cup	18.00
Papayas, raw	1 papaya	17.94
Watermelon, raw	1 wedge	17.73
Yogurt, plain, skim milk	8-oz. container	17.43
Honey	1 Tbsp.	17.25
Ice cream, chocolate	½ cup	16.74
Cereal, Quaker, low-fat granola	½ cup	16.71
Fruit leather, pieces	1 oz.	16.32
Pears, raw	1 pear	16.27
Prunes, uncooked	5 prunes	16.01
Milk chocolate coated peanuts	10 pieces	15.04
Carob candies	1 oz.	14.74

DESCRIPTION	MEASURE	CONTENT/MEASURE (G)
Blueberries, raw	1 cup	14.44
Bananas, raw	1 banana	14.43
Jerusalem artichokes, raw	1 cup	14.40
Pineapple, raw	1 cup	14.35
Apples, raw, with skin	1 apple	14.34
Peaches, raw	1 cup	14.26
Doughnuts, yeast leavened, glazed	1 medium	14.23
Ice cream, vanilla	½ cup	14.01
Melons, honeydew, raw	⅛ melon	12.99
Milk, whole,	1 cup	12.83
Fruitcake, commercially prepared	1 piece	12.83
Milk, low fat, 1 percent milk fat	1 cup	12.69
Milk, nonfat, (fat free or skim)	1 cup	12.47
Milk, reduced fat, 2 percent milk fat	1 cup	12.35
Sweet potato, baked in skin	1 potato	12.32
Orange, raw	1 orange	12.25
Milk, dry, nonfat, instant	⅓ cup	12.00
Maple syrup	1 Tbsp.	11.90
Buttermilk, low fat	1 cup	11.74
Toaster pastries, fruit	1 pastry	11.36

DESCRIPTION	MEASURE	CONTENT/MEASURE (G)
Tomatoes, canned, stewed	1 cup	11.25
Nectarine, raw	1 nectarine	10.73
Doughnuts, cake type, plain	1 medium	10.58
Tomato sauce, canned	1 cup	10.41
Jellies	1 Tbsp.	9.73
Jams and preserves	1 Tbsp.	9.70
Onions, boiled, drained	1 cup	9.51
Lettuce, iceberg, raw	1 head	9.49
Watermelon, raw	1 cup	9.42
Chocolate syrup	1 Tbsp.	9.31
Carrot juice, canned	1 cup	9.23
Tangerine, raw	1 tangerine	8.89
Cherries, sweet, raw	10 cherries	8.72
Tomato juice, canned	1 cup	8.65
Grapefruit, raw, white	½ grapefruit	8.63
Grapefruit, raw, pink and red	½ grapefruit	8.47
Raisins, seedless	1 packet	8.29
Pineapple, canned, heavy syrup	1 slice	8.28
Peaches, raw	1 peach	8.22

DESCRIPTION	MEASURE	CONTENT/MEASURE (G)
Pumpkin, canned	1 cup	8.09
Vegetable juice cocktail, canned	1 cup	7.99
Chickpeas (garbanzos), boiled	1 cup	7.87
Sugar, powdered	1 Tbsp.	7.83
Grapes, red or green, raw	10 grapes	7.74
Strawberries, raw	1 cup	7.74
Cookies, fig bars	1 cookie	7.42
Orange juice, raw	juice from 1 orange	7.22
Blackberries, raw	1 cup	7.03
Onions, raw	1 cup	6.85
Kiwi fruit, raw	1 medium	6.83
Pineapple, canned, juice pack	1 slice	6.79
Squash, winter, baked	1 cup	6.77
Pancake syrup, table blend	1 Tbsp.	6.62
Caramel candies	1 piece	6.62
Plums, raw	1 plum	6.55
Croissant, butter	1 croissant	6.42
Peas, edible pods, boiled, drained	1 cup	6.38

DESCRIPTION	MEASURE	CONTENT/MEASURE (G)
Milk chocolate coated raisins	10 pieces	6.22
Oatmeal cookie, commercial,	1 cookie, regular	6.17
Tomatoes, canned, whole	1 cup	6.14
Vanilla sandwich cookie	1 cookie	5.90
Molasses cookie	1 cookie, large (3½" to 4")	5.63
Lima beans, large, boiled	1 cup	5.45
Raspberries, raw	1 cup	5.44
Carrots, boiled, drained	1 cup	5.38
Cottage cheese with fruit	1 cup	5.38
Corn syrup, light	1 Tbsp.	5.35
Soybeans, mature, boiled,	1 cup	5.16
Cucumber, with peel, raw	1 large	5.03
Peppers, sweet, red, raw	1 pepper	5.00
Carrots, raw	1 cup	4.99
Cookies, peanut butter, commercial	1 cookie, regular	4.77
General Mills Whole Grain Total	¾ cup	4.73
Kellogg's All-Bran	½ cup	4.71

DESCRIPTION	MEASURE	CONTENT/MEASURE (G)
Muffin, oat bran	1 muffin	4.69
Turnips, boiled, drained	1 cup	4.66
Squash, summer, boiled, drained	1 cup	4.66
Kohlrabi, boiled, drained	1 cup	4.62
Bagels, plain, enriched	4" bagel	4.49
Cabbage, boiled, drained	1 cup	4.38
Hoisin sauce, ready to serve	1 Tbsp.	4.36
Mung beans, sprouted, raw	1 cup	4.30
Miso	1 cup	4.26
General Mills Wheaties	1 cup	4.20
Sugar, granulated	1 tsp.	4.20
Fast food, pepperoni, regular crust	1 slice, 14" pizza	4.04
Kellogg's Special K	1 cup	4.00
Kellogg's Product 19	1 cup	3.99
Beets, boiled, drained	1 beet	3.98
Okra, boiled, drained	1 cup	3.84
Hard candy	1 piece	3.77
Carambola (star fruit), raw	1 fruit	3.62

DESCRIPTION	MEASURE	CONTENT/MEASURE (G)
Sugar cookie, refrigerator, baked	1 cookie	3.59
Russian salad dressing, low calorie	1 Tbsp.	3.56
Lentils, boiled	1 cup	3.56
Mushrooms, canned, drained	1 cup	3.43
Ketchup	1 Tbsp.	3.42
Lime juice, unsweetened	1 cup	3.37
Russian salad dressing	1 Tbsp.	3.31
Carrot, raw	1 carrot	3.27
Tomatoes, red, ripe, raw	1 tomato	3.23
Apricot, raw	1 apricot	3.23
Buckwheat flour, whole groat	1 cup	3.12
Brown sugar	1 tsp.	3.08
Peppers, sweet, green, raw	1 pepper	2.86
Cabbage, red, raw	1 cup	2.74
Brussels sprouts, boiled, drained	1 cup	2.71
Rolls, hamburger or hot dog, plain	1 roll	2.69
Bread, mixed grain	1 slice	2.61
French salad dressing, reduced fat	1 Tbsp.	2.60

DESCRIPTION	MEASURE	CONTENT/MEASURE (G)
French salad dressing, regular	1 Tbsp.	2.49
Lima beans, frozen, baby, boiled	1 cup	2.47
Corn, sweet, yellow, boiled, drained	1 ear	2.44
Cauliflower, raw	1 cup	2.40
Pickle relish, sweet	1 Tbsp.	2.40
Peppers, hot chili, red, raw	1 pepper	2.39
Potato, baked, flesh and skin	1 potato	2.38
Pancake syrup, table, low calorie	1 Tbsp.	2.32
Peppers, hot chili, green, raw	1 pepper	2.30
Pickles, cucumber, dill	1 pickle	2.28
English muffins, plain, toasted	1 muffin	1.80
Cream substitute (oil, soy protein)	1 Tbsp.	1.71
Artichokes, boiled, drained	1 cup	1.66
Beans, yellow, boiled, drained	1 cup	1.66
Beans, green, boiled, drained	1 cup	1.66
Waffles, plain, ready to eat	1 waffle	1.66

DESCRIPTION	MEASURE	CONTENT/MEASURE (G)
Pretzels, hard, plain, salted	10 pretzels	1.66
Broccoli, raw	1 cup	1.50
Peanut butter, smooth	1 Tbsp.	1.48
Lemons, raw, without peel	1 lemon	1.45
Cashew nuts	1 oz. (18 nuts)	1.42
Almonds	1 oz. (24 nuts)	1.36
Nuts, hazelnuts or filberts	1 oz.	1.23
Soy milk	1 cup	1.23
Peanuts, all types	1 oz. (approx 28)	1.19
Potato chips, plain, salted	1 oz.	1.17
Feta cheese	1 oz.	1.16
Mushrooms, raw	1 cup	1.16
Crackers, wheat, regular	4 crackers	1.04
Bread, white, commercial	1 slice	1.04
Kellogg's Eggo low-fat waffle	1 waffle	1.02
Pine nuts, dried	1 oz.	1.02
Bread, rye	1 slice	1.02
Rolls, hard (includes kaiser)	1 roll	1.01
Soup, beef bouillon, dry powder	1 packet	1.00
Spinach, boiled, drained	1 cup	0.97

DESCRIPTION	MEASURE	CONTENT/MEASURE (G)
Cornmeal, whole grain, yellow	1 cup	0.78
Asparagus, boiled, drained	4 spears	0.78
Pita bread, white	6½ pita	0.78
Walnuts, English	1 oz. (14 halves)	0.74
Celery, raw	1 stalk	0.73
Brown rice, long grain, cooked	1 cup	0.68
Oats, all types, cooked	1 cup	0.56
Egg, whole, hard boiled	1 large	0.56
Butter	1 Tbsp.	0.01
Club soda	12 fl oz.	0.00
Teas	6–8 oz. cup	0.00
Coffees	6–8 oz. cup	0.00
Meats braised, broiled, roasted, fried	any size serving	0.00

PRODUCT SOURCES

C ONSIDER ONE OR more of the following recommended products to address your mood-related concerns:

DR. JANET'S BALANCED BY NATURE PRODUCTS

These products are available by calling (800) 231-8485.

Tranquility

GABA Stress Formula—Promotes a feeling of well-being for the body and mind.

$21.95

Each three capsules contain:

- GABA, 500 mg
- Glycine, 250 mg
- Cramp bark powder, 200 mg
- Dong quai, 150 mg
- Passionflower, 250 mg
- Vitamin B_6, 50 mg
- Magnesium (citrate), 16 mg

GABA and glycine (natural tranquilizers) are calmatives for nerve impulses, controlling muscle contractions. Both are inhibitory neurotransmitters.

Cramp bark has been used historically for alleviating muscle pain related to exercise, stress, or physical activity.

Dong quai root extract has been used for centuries in Chinese traditional health practice. Dong quai functions to increase the relaxation of smooth muscles.

Passionflower has a sedative, calmative effect.

B_6 is the "antistress" vitamin.

Magnesium helps prevent depression, dizziness, muscle weakness, twitching, heart disease and high blood pressure, irritability and nervousness.

Safe Passage

For women in the perimenopause and menopause stage of life. $24.95

Each two capsules contain:

- Black cohosh root extract, 160 mg
- Protykin, 8 mg
- Licorice root extract, 75 mg
- Gamma oryzanol, 300 mg
- Dong quai root extract, 75 mg

Black cohosh is a powerful phytoestrogen that binds to hormone receptors in the uterus, breast, and other parts of the body, lessening hot flashes, vaginal dryness, headache, dizziness, depressive mood, and other hormone-related symptoms. Used in Europe since the nineteenth century, the use of black cohosh has been backed up by over forty years of clinical research.

Protykin is the same dietary phytoestrogen found in grapes and red wines. Its unique structure allows for estrogenic and antiestrogenic activities while also providing cardioprotective effects.

Licorice helps enhance estrogen levels. Licorice has estrogen- and progesterone-like effects. It helps reduce spasms, helps stimulate the production of interferon, and may stimulate natural defense mechanisms that increase the amount of mucus-secreting cells in the gastrointestinal tract.

Dong quai enhances the effect of ovarian hormones. It is used to treat vaginal dryness, PMS, hot flashes, and other menopausal symptoms. It has ginseng properties that balance female hormones, improve circulation, relieve stress, and purify and strengthen blood.

Women's Balance Formula (Progesterone Cream)

For women who experience mood swings, lack of energy, depression, cramps, migraines, and other symptoms related to PMS and menopause. Progesterone cream helps to balance the symptoms of estrogen dominance that affect so many women today. It is formulated to match the physiological amount of progesterone needed to maintain a woman's balance.

$24.95

Everyone is different. The use of progesterone cream should be adjusted to meet your own needs. The following suggestions are to be used as a guide only. Although there have been no reports of any significant side effects or health problems associated with the use of this progesterone cream, you may consider consulting your health-care provider. Results vary from woman to woman. Some notice changes immediately, while others see changes in one to three months.

For PMS and perimenopausal symptoms:

- After ovulation (days 14–18 after onset of last period)— use no more than ¼ tsp. once daily.

- Day 18–23—use ¼ tsp. twice daily, gradually increasing to ½ tsp. twice daily.

- Day 23 until period starts—use ½ tsp. twice daily.

For osteoporosis:

- Use ¼ tsp. (½ tsp. for severe cases) daily. (Before using this formula, bone density testing is recommended to determine a base line from which to measure the changes in your bone density every six to twelve months. Consult your health-care provider.)

For postmenopausal women:

- Use cream for three weeks, ¼–½ tsp. twice per day. Then go one week without applying the cream.

Dr. Janet's Glucosamine Cream

Glucosamine cream provides quick topical relief to inflamed joints and sore muscles caused by overwork, daily activity, or arthritis. Glucosamine cream contains and works with the body's natural hormones to provide quick, safe, pain relief. If used regularly, it can act as a preventive measure.

Glucosamine cream includes a high-quality formulation of emu oil, pregnenolone, and glucosamine sulfate, along with proper amounts of specially selected herbs, vitamins, and enzymes.

$24.95

PAIN AND STRESS CENTER PRODUCTS

For more information on amino-acid formulas or to order, contact:

The Pain and Stress Center

(800) 669-2256

http://www.painstresscenter.com

Pain and Stress Center products include:

- Brain Link
- Anxiety Control 24

NOTES

CHAPTER 1
THE MIND-BODY CONNECTION

1. Candace Pert, "Emotional Stress Leads to Immune Suppression," *Prevention,* April 1994, 73–79.

2. From the Bodyworks food and fitness journals, published by the National Women's Health Information Center, U.S. Department of Health and Human Services, Office on Women's Health, http://www.4women.gov/bodyworks/toolkit (accessed November 2, 2007).

3. "Emotional Wrecks," *Health,* January/February 1999, 70.

4. Adapted from "When Unwanted Thoughts Take Over: Obsessive-Compulsive Disorder," a booklet published in 2007 by the National Institute of Mental Health. Free information available at http://www.nimh.nih.gov/health/publications/when-unwanted-thoughts-take-over-obsessive-compulsive-disorder/obsessive-compulsive-disorder.shtml (accessed November 14, 2007).

5. Reprinted from "Post-Traumatic Stress Disorder, A Real Illness," a booklet published in 2005 by the National Institute of Mental Health. Free information available at http://www.nimh.nih.gov/health/publications/post-traumatic-stress-disorder-a-real-illness/summary.shtml (accessed November 14, 2007).

6. From "Panic Disorder, A Real Illness," a booklet published in 2006 by the National Institute of Mental Health. Free information available at http://www.nimh.nih.gov/health/publications/panic-disorder-a-real-illness/summary.shtml (accessed November 14, 2007).

7. Suggestions taken from results of The Food and Mood Project survey, a study undertaken in Great Britain with the support of a Millennium Award from "Mind," a mental health charity in the United Kingdom, and the Cyril Cordon Trust. Survey results at www.foodandmood.org/Pages/sh-survey.html (accessed November 14, 2007). The Food and Mood Project, P.O. Box 2737, Lewes, East Sussex, BN7 2GN, U.K.

CHAPTER 2
HORMONES AND YOUR DIET

1. USDA Database for the Flavonoid Content of Selected Foods, Release 2.1 (2007), United States Department of Agriculture, http://www.nal.usda.gov/fnic/foodcomp/Data/Flav/Flav02-1.pdf (accessed November 14, 2007).

2. John R. Lee, MD, with Jesse Hanley and Virginia Hopkins, *What Your Doctor May Not Tell You About Perimenopause* (New York: Warner Books, 1999), 60.

3. U.S. Department of Agriculture, Dietary Guidelines for Americans 2005, http://www.health.gov/dietaryguidelines/dga2005/document/default.htm (accessed November 14, 2007). Nutrient values from Agricultural Research Service (ARS) Nutrient Database for Standard Reference, Release 17.

4. R. D. Mattes and D. Donnelly, "Relative Contributions of Dietary Sodium Sources." *Journal of the American College of Nutrition*, 10, no. 4 (August 10, 1991): 383–393.

5. Adapted from "Healthy Menopause Diet—15 Suggestions," Anne Collins Weight Loss Program, http://www.annecollins.com/best-diet-for-menopause.htm (accessed November 14, 2007).

CHAPTER 3
STRESS AND YOUR DIET

1. Adapted from Terry Farris, "Anti-Stress Diet," iVillage.co.uk, http://www.ivillage.co.uk/food/experts/coach/articles/0,,177274_601071,00.html (accessed November 14, 2007).

CHAPTER 4
FATIGUE AND YOUR DIET

1. Linda Rector Page, "Sugar and Substitutes: Are They All Bad?" *Healthy Healing—A Guide to Self-Healing for Everyone* (Carmel Valley, CA: 2000), 69.

2. "Special Diets for Food Allergies," Cleveland Clinic Foundation health information resources, http://www.clevelandclinic.org/health/health-info/docs/2900/2987.asp?index=10014.

3. Ibid.

CHAPTER 5
DEPRESSION AND YOUR DIET

1. Harvard School of Public Health, "What Is Protein?" http://www.hsph.harvard.edu/nutritionsource/protein.html (accessed November 15, 2007).

2. Ibid.

3. Ibid.

4. Susan E. Gebhardt and Robin G. Thomas, "Nutritive Value of Foods," United States Department of Agriculture (USDA), http://www.nal.usda.gov/fnic/foodcomp/Data/HG72/hg72_2002 .pdf (accessed December 28, 2007).

5. Medline Plus Medical Encyclopedia, a service of the U.S. National Library of Medicine and the National Institutes of Health, http://www.nlm.nih.gov/medlineplus/ency.

CHAPTER 6
THE FEEL-GOOD DIET PROGRAM

1. Joseph Hibbeln, MD, lead clinical investigator for the National Institute on Alcohol Abuse and Alcoholism, Bethesda, MD.

2. John R. Lee, MD, *What Your Doctor May Not Tell You About Menopause* (New York, Warner Books, 1996).

3. Elizabeth Somer, *Food & Mood*, as quoted by Charles Stuart Platkin in "Change in Your Mood? It Just Might Be Your Food," *Honolulu Advertiser*, July 16, 2003; archived at http://the .honoluluadvertiser.com/article/2003/Jul/16/il/il07a (accessed August 10, 2007).

4. Gebhardt and Thomas, "Nutritive Value of Foods."

APPENDIX A
FOOD SOURCES FOR SELECTED VITAMINS, MINERALS, AND OTHER NUTRIENTS

1. U.S. Department of Agriculture, Dietary Guidelines for Americans 2005 http://www.health.gov/dietaryguidelines/ dga2005/document/default.htm (accessed November 16, 2007). Nutrient values from Agricultural Research Service (ARS) Nutrient Database for Standard Reference, Release 17. Foods are from ARS single nutrient reports, sorted in descending order by nutrient content in terms of common household measures. Food items and weights in the single nutrient reports are adapted from those in 2002 revision of USDA Home and Garden Bulletin No. 72, Nutritive Value of Foods. Mixed dishes and multiple preparations of the same food item have been omitted from this table.

2. Ibid.

3. Ibid.

4. U.S. Department of Agriculture, Agricultural Research Service, 2005. USDA National Nutrient Database for Standard Reference, Release 18. Nutrient Data Laboratory home page, http://www .ars.usda.gov/ba/bhnrc/ndl (accessed November 16, 2007).

5. Ibid.

6. U.S. Department of Agriculture, Dietary Guidelines for Americans 2005, http://www.health.gov/dietaryguidelines/ dga2005/document/default.htm (accessed November 16, 2007). Nutrient values from Agricultural Research Service (ARS) Nutrient Database for Standard Reference, Release 17. Foods are from ARS single nutrient reports, sorted in descending order by nutrient content in terms of common household measures. Food items and weights in the single nutrient reports are adapted from those in 2002 revision of USDA Home and Garden Bulletin No. 72, Nutritive Value of Foods. Mixed dishes and multiple preparations of the same food item have been omitted from this table.

7. Ibid.

8. Ibid.

9. U.S. Department of Agriculture, Agricultural Research Service. 2005. USDA National Nutrient Database for Standard Reference, Release 18. Nutrient Data Laboratory home page, http://www .ars.usda.gov/ba/bhnrc/ndl (accessed November 16, 2007).

10. ARS Nutrient Database for Standard Reference, Release 17. Foods are from single nutrient reports, which are sorted either by food description or in descending order by nutrient content in terms of common household measures. The food items and weights in these reports are adapted from those in 2002 revision of USDA Home and Garden Bulletin No. 72, Nutritive Value of Foods. Mixed dishes and multiple preparations of the same food item have been omitted.

11. U.S. Department of Agriculture, Dietary Guidelines for Americans 2005, http://www.health.gov/dietaryguidelines/ dga2005/document/default.htm (accessed November 16, 2007). Nutrient values from Agricultural Research Service (ARS) Nutrient Database for Standard Reference, Release 17. Foods are from ARS single nutrient reports, sorted in descending order by nutrient content in terms of common household measures. Food items and weights in the single nutrient reports are adapted from those in 2002 revision of USDA Home and Garden Bulletin No. 72, Nutritive Value of Foods. Mixed dishes and multiple preparations of the same food item have been omitted from this table.

12. U.S. Department of Agriculture, Agricultural Research Service. 2005. USDA National Nutrient Database for Standard Reference, Release 18. Nutrient Data Laboratory home page, http://www .ars.usda.gov/ba/bhnrc/ndl (accessed November 16, 2007).

Experience
Better Health
in all Areas of Your Life Today!

We hope that you have discovered delicious new ways to improve your emotional health. Here are two more books by Janet Maccaro that will help you look and feel great in the years to come.

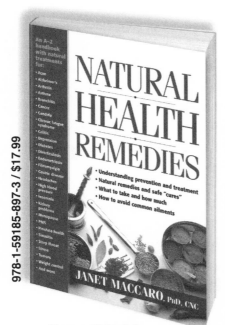

978-1-59185-897-3 / $17.99

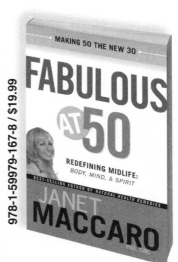

978-1-59979-167-8 / $19.99

Natural Health Remedies

Arm yourself with the health tips and tools you need to be renewed and restored to good health naturally!

Fabulous at 50

Learn how to turn back the clock on aging with this fact-filled, inspirational book. Make your fifties—and beyond—the best years of your life!

7718 Visit your local bookstore today!

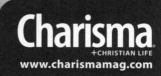